W9-BUI-203

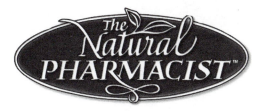

The
Natural
PHARMACIST™

Your Complete Guide to Illnesses and Their Natural Remedies

Steven Bratman, M.D.

Series Editors

Steven Bratman, M.D.
& David Kroll, Ph.D.

Prima
HEALTH

A DIVISION OF PRIMA PUBLISHING

Visit us online at www.primahealth.com

PRIMA HEALTH and colophon are trademarks of Prima Communications, Inc.
THE NATURAL PHARMACIST™ is a trademark of Prima Communications, Inc.

All products mentioned in this book are trademarks of their respective companies.

Library of Congress Cataloging-in-Publication Data

Bratman, Steven.
 Your Complete Guide to Illnesses and Their Natural Remedies / Steven Bratman.
  p.   cm.—(The natural pharmacist)
 Includes bibliographical references and index.
 ISBN 0-7615-1791-X
 1. Herbs—Therapeutic use. 2. Dietary supplements. I. Title. II. Series.
RM666.H33B7244 1999
615.'321—dc21   98-43896
                                                                         CIP

99 00 01 02 HH 10 9 8 7 6 5 4 3 2 1
Printed in the United States of America

Visit us online at www.thenaturalpharmacist.com

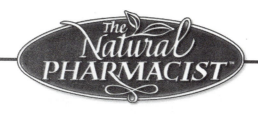

Inside—Find the Answers to These Questions and More

☑ How can echinacea, andrographis, zinc, vitamin C, elderberry, and ginkgo help colds and flus? (See page 92.)

☑ Can ginkgo, phosphatidylserine, and L-acetyl-carnitine improve memory and mental function? (See page 5.)

☑ Can a combination of vitamins E and C help prevent atherosclerosis? (See page 30.)

☑ What is ipriflavone and how can it help prevent or treat osteoporosis? (See page 212.)

☑ If I have diabetes, can chromium help control my blood sugar levels? (See page 128.)

☑ What can I do to reduce nausea during pregnancy? (See page 194.)

☑ By what percentage can garlic lower my high blood pressure levels? (See page 158.)

☑ What can I do to reduce the agony of migraine headaches? (See page 184.)

☑ How can I reduce the discomfort of varicose veins? (See page 235.)

☑ Can chondroitin sulfate actually slow the progression of osteoarthritis? (See page 202.)

THE NATURAL PHARMACIST Library

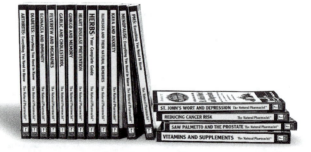

Contents

Contents

What Makes This Book Different?

The interest in natural medicine has never been greater. According to the National Association of Chain Drug Stores, 65 million Americans are using natural supplements, and the number is growing! Yet, it is hard for the consumer to find trustworthy sources for balanced information about this emerging field. Why? Frankly, natural medicine has had a checkered history. From snake oil potions sold at the turn of the century to those books, magazines, and product catalogs that hype miracle cures today, this is a field where exaggerated claims have been the norm. Proponents of natural medicine have tended to abuse science, treating it more as a marketing tool than a means of discovering the truth.

But there is truth to be found. Studies of vitamins, minerals, and other food supplements have been with us since these nutritional substances were first discovered, and the level and quality of this science has grown dramatically in the last 20 years. Herbal medicine has been neglected in the United States, but in Europe, this, the oldest of all healing arts, has been the subject of tremendous and ongoing scientific interest.

At present, for a number of herbs and supplements, it is possible to give reasonably scientific answers to the questions: "How well does this work? How safe is it? What types of conditions is it best used for?"

THE NATURAL PHARMACIST series is designed to cut through the hype and tell you what we know and what we don't know about popular natural treatments. These books are more conservative than any others available, more honest about the weaknesses of natural approaches, more fair in their comparisons of natural and conventional treatments. You won't find any miracle cures here; but you will discover useful options that can help you become healthier.

Why Choose Natural Treatments?

Although the science behind natural medicine continues to grow, this is still a much less scientifically validated field than conventional medicine. You might ask, "Why should I resort to an herb that is only partly proven, when I could take a drug with solid science behind it?" There are at least three good reasons to consider natural alternatives.

First, some herbs and supplements offer benefits that are not matched by any conventional drug. Vitamin E is a good example. It appears to help prevent prostate cancer, a benefit that no standard medication can claim. Also, vitamin E almost certainly helps prevent heart disease. While there are standard drugs that also prevent heart disease, vitamin E works differently and may be able to complement many of the other approaches.

Another example is the herb milk thistle. Studies strongly suggest that this herb can protect the liver from injury. There is no pill or tablet your doctor can prescribe to do the same.

Even if the science behind some of these treatments is less than perfect, when the risks are low and the possible benefit high, a treatment may be worth trying. It is a little known fact that for many conventional treatments the science is less than perfect as well, and physicians must balance uncertain benefits against incompletely understood risks.

A second reason to consider natural therapies is that some may offer benefits comparable to those of drugs with fewer side effects. The herb St. John's wort is a good example. Reasonably strong scientific evidence suggests that this herb is an effective treatment for mild to moderate depression, while producing fewer side effects on average than conventional medications. Saw palmetto for benign enlargement of the prostate, ginkgo for relieving symptoms and perhaps slowing the progression of Alzheimer's disease, and glucosamine for osteoarthritis are other examples. This is not to say that herbs and supplements are completely harmless—they're not—but for most the level of risk is quite low.

Finally, there is a philosophical point to consider. For many people, it "feels" better to use a treatment that comes from nature instead of from a laboratory. Just as you might rather wear all-cotton clothing than polyester, or look at a mountain landscape rather than the skyscrapers of a downtown city, natural treatments may simply feel more compatible with your view of life. We can quibble endlessly about just what "natural" means and whether a certain treatment is "actually" natural or not, but such arguments are beside the point. The difference is in the feeling, and feelings matter. In fact, having a good feeling about taking an herb may lead you to use it more consistently than you would a prescription drug

Of course, at times synthetic drugs may be necessary and even lifesaving. But on many other occasions it may be quite reasonable to turn to an herb or supplement instead of a drug.

To make good decisions you need good information. Unfortunately, while hundreds of books on alternative medicine are published every year, many are highly misleading. The phrase "studies prove" is often used when the studies in question are so small or so badly conducted that they prove nothing at all. You may even find that the "data" from other books comes from studies with petri dishes and not real people!

You can't even assume that books written by well-known authors are scientifically sound. Many of these authors rely on secondary writers, leading to a game of "telephone" where misconceptions are passed around from book to book. And there's a strong tendency to exaggerate the power of natural remedies, whitewashing them with selective reporting.

THE NATURAL PHARMACIST series gives you the balanced information you need to make informed decisions about your health needs. Setting a new, high standard of accuracy and objectivity, these books take a realistic look at the herbs and supplements you read about in the news. You will encounter both favorable and unfavorable studies in these pages and will learn about both the benefits and the risks of natural treatments.

THE NATURAL PHARMACIST series is the source you can trust.

Steven Bratman, M.D.
David Kroll, Ph.D.

Introduction

What we don't know about health and illness vastly exceeds what we do know. Over the centuries, numerous methods of healing have been invented, but they are all based on partial knowledge. Healing illnesses is simply a lot more difficult than, say, fixing cars. Not only is the human body enormously more complex than an automobile, it doesn't come with an owner's manual. We can learn how cars work because people invented them, but since we were not privy to the design of the human body we have to start from scratch.

The problem of discovering what works in healing is made even more complex by the influence of the mind. Numerous scientific studies have shown that sugar pills can produce dramatically beneficial effects in up to 50 or 60% of the individuals who take them. Placebo treatment not only relieves headaches, improves urination, and reduces pain but it can also alter blood pressure, cholesterol levels, and the microscopic appearance of cells. This simply does not happen with cars. If you turn a wrench and the engine runs better, you can be pretty sure it wasn't the power of suggestion. But if you try an herb or a drug and notice an improvement in your symptoms, you can't be so sure that it was specifically the herb or drug that made the difference.

Over the last century, conventional medicine gradually evolved an elegant method of getting around the placebo effect. The so-called double-blind placebo-controlled study allows us to be more certain than ever before in history that a treatment actually accomplishes its immediate goals. In such a study, half the participants receive real treatment, the other half placebo treatment, but neither the patient nor the doctor knows who is receiving which one. This eliminates the power of suggestion from two directions. Not only is the influence of suggestion on the patient factored out, a double-blind study also protects the doctor from bias based on expectation.

By using double-blind studies and other careful scientific techniques, conventional medicine has gained society's confidence and become the dominant health-care system worldwide. Yet for a reason that is more practical than scientific, certain forms of treatment have been neglected. It is expensive to perform double-blind studies, and by and large, the source of money for such studies comes from manufacturers of products for which they hold a patent.

Treatments like herbs and vitamins, on the other hand, are not patentable and as a result simply don't have as obvious a source of funds for scientific investigation, even for good double-blind testing. In addition, since numerous manufacturers sell the same types of herbs, no one manufacturer is willing to invest money in expensive studies that will serve to also benefit the competition. Therefore, they have remained largely outside the mainstream, falling in the realm of alternative medicine. (Other obstacles have also caused difficulties in these treatments' incorporation into mainstream medicine. For more information on this interesting subject, see *The Natural Pharmacist: Your Complete Guide to Herbs* and *The Natural Pharmacist: Your Complete Guide to Vitamins and Supplements.*)

This exclusion of certain treatments has been unfortunate for consumers, who would like to make use of all their health-care options regardless of the flow of research dollars. Fortunately, in recent years the level of scientific investigation into herbs and supplements has grown tremendously. There has also been a migration of knowledge from Europe and other countries where double-blind studies of herbs and supplements are somewhat easier to fund.

This book summarizes the best-documented herb and supplement treatments for over 50 conditions. There are many other illnesses for which herbs and supplements are rumored to work, but this book only covers those for which there are natural treatments with at least some substantial evidence of effectiveness. This is not to say that the treatments in this book are solidly proven. Research into natural options is still a work in progress, and we do not yet have all the documentation we'd like. In some cases, the evidence is surprisingly good; in others, it's weaker than some media reporting would have you believe. Like all THE NATURAL PHARMACIST books, this one analyzes the research evidence fairly to give you a sense of how securely you can trust the results.

Please remember that no book can substitute for individualized medical attention. Every person is different and has specific health needs only a health-care practitioner can address. Furthermore, in many cases it is possible to use combinations of treatments in a more sophisticated fashion than can be presented here. The information contained in the following chapters should be regarded as an introduction, a suggestion for where to start.

ACNE

The blackheads and sometimes painful pimples that we know as acne occur most commonly during adolescence, but they may persist into later life as well. There is much we still don't understand about what causes acne. We do know that during adolescence and other times of hormonal imbalance, such as around menopause, the oil-secreting glands in the skin increase their level of secretions. A combination of naturally occurring yeast and bacteria then breaks down these secretions, causing the skin to become inflamed and the pimples to eventually rupture. In severe cases, acne can lead to permanent scars.

Conventional treatment, which usually is quite successful, consists primarily of antibiotics, cleansing agents, and chemically modified versions of vitamin A.

Natural Treatments for Acne

While there are no dramatically effective alternative treatments for acne, there are a few options that may provide some help.

Warning: Do not rely on any of the treatments discussed in this section to treat severe acne where scarring is a consideration.

Zinc

People with acne have been shown to have lower-than-normal levels of zinc in their bodies.[1–4] However, this doesn't prove that taking zinc supplements will help acne. For example, it is possible that the factors that cause acne also affect zinc levels.

Double-blind studies involving a total of more than 300 people have tried to discover whether taking extra zinc can relieve the symptoms of acne. The results have been generally positive, indicating a definite but somewhat mild effect.

In one double-blind study of 54 people, oral zinc produced a noticeable improvement in about one-third of those who received it.[5] The results of other studies have been similarly modest.[6–10] One study found that zinc was as effective as a tetracycline-type of antibiotic;[11] but another found that tetracycline was more effective,[12] which is usually the case in real life.

A typical dosage of zinc is 30 mg daily as zinc citrate or gluconate, combined with 1 to 3 mg daily of supplemental copper. Too much zinc can be toxic, so it is important not to exceed this dosage. The beneficial effects take 12 weeks to develop.

Other Herbs and Supplements

Other commonly mentioned natural treatments for acne include chromium, vitamin E, vitamin B_6, selenium, burdock, and red clover. Tea tree oil has antiseptic properties and has been suggested as an alternative to benzoyl peroxide for direct application to the skin. There haven't been any solid studies examining these treatments, however.

ALLERGIES
(Hay Fever)

(For Other Types of Allergies, see Asthma and Eczema)

Principal Natural Treatments
There are no well-established natural treatments for allergies.

Other Natural Treatments
Nettle, flavonoids, vitamin C, B vitamins

About 7% of all Americans suffer from hay fever, an allergic condition that can cause runny nose, sneezing, and teary eyes. It is known officially as *allergic rhinitis, allergic sinusitis,* or *allergic conjunctivitis,* depending on whether symptoms manifest mainly in the nose, sinuses, or eyes, respectively. Hay fever usually peaks when particular plants are pollinating or when molds are flourishing. People who suffer from year-round hay fever may be allergic to ever-present allergens such as dust mites.

Here's how hay fever works. In response to the triggers noted above, an individual prone to allergies develops an exaggerated immune response. Substances known as IgEs flood the nasal passages, white blood cells called eosinophils arrive by the millions and billions, and inflammatory substances such as histamine, prostaglandins, and leukotrienes are released in massive amounts. The overall effect is the familiar one of swelling, dripping, itching, and aching.

The mechanism of allergic response is fairly well understood. Why allergic people react so excessively to innocent bits of pollen, however, remains a complete mystery.

Conventional treatment for hay fever consists of antihistamines (now available in forms that don't make you sleepy); decongestants, nasal steroids, or cromolyn sodium; and occasionally allergic desensitization ("allergy shots"). For most people, some combination of these treatments will be successful.

Natural Treatments for Allergies

The following treatments are widely recommended for allergies, but they have not been scientifically proven effective at this time.

Nettle Leaf

According to one preliminary double-blind study, freeze-dried extract of stinging nettle leaf can help improve allergy symptoms.[1]

A typical dosage is two to three 300-mg capsules of nettle leaf. Nettle leaf has an extensive history of use in food and is believed to be safe. However, safety in young children, pregnant or nursing women, and those with severe liver or kidney disease has not been established.

For theoretical reasons, some researchers suggest that nettle may interact with conventional medications for diabetes and high blood pressure, but no actual problems of this type have been officially reported.

Flavonoids

Test-tube studies suggest that flavonoids—biologically active compounds found in many plants—may help reduce allergy symptoms.[2–5] A particular flavonoid, quercetin, seems to be one of the most active.[6–10] Many texts on natural medicine claim that quercetin works like the drug cromolyn (Intal) by stopping the release of allergenic substances in the body. However, while we have direct evidence that cromolyn is effective, there have not been any published studies in which people were given quercetin and their allergic symptoms decreased. It is a long way from test-tube studies to real people. At the present time, we don't really know whether taking quercetin or other flavonoids is helpful for allergies. If you do wish to take quercetin, a particular form of the substance, *quercetin chalcone,* may be better absorbed than other forms.

Vitamin C

Vitamin C is often suggested as a treatment for allergies, but it does not appear to work. Of the double-blind studies that have been performed, more have found it ineffective than effective.[11,12,13]

B Vitamins

Vitamins B_6 and B_{12} are often recommended for hay fever. Again, there is no significant evidence that they are effective.

ALZHEIMER'S DISEASE
(and Non-Alzheimer's Dementia)

Principal Natural Treatments
Ginkgo, phosphatidylserine, L-acetyl-carnitine

Other Natural Treatments
Vitamin E, vitamin C, phosphatidylcholine, zinc, magnesium, DHEA, vitamin B_{12}

Alzheimer's disease is the most common cause of progressive mental deterioration (dementia) in the elderly. It has been estimated that 30 to 50% of people over 85 years old suffer from this disease.

Microscopic examination shows that nerve cells in the thinking parts of the brain have died and disappeared, particularly cells that release a chemical called acetylcholine. However, we do not know exactly what causes Alzheimer's disease.

Alzheimer's begins with subtle symptoms, such as loss of memory for names and recent events. It progresses from difficulty learning new information, to a few eccentric behaviors, to depression, loss of spontaneity, and anxiety. Over the course of the disease, the individual gradually loses the ability to carry out the activities of everyday life. Disorientation, asking questions repeatedly, and an inability to recognize friends are characteristics of moderately severe Alzheimer's. Eventually, virtually all mental functions fail.

Similar symptoms may be caused by conditions other than Alzheimer's disease, such as multiple small strokes (called multi-infarct dementia), alcoholism, and certain rarer causes. It is very important to begin with an examination to discover what is causing the symptoms of mental decline. Various easily treatable conditions, such as depression, can mimic the symptoms of dementia.

Once the diagnosis of Alzheimer's or non-Alzheimer's dementia has been made, treatment may begin with drugs such as Cognex or Aricept. These medications usually produce a modest improvement in mild to moderate Alzheimer's disease by increasing the duration of action of acetylcholine. However, they can cause sometimes severe side effects due to the exaggeration of acetylcholine's action in other parts of the body.

Principal Natural Treatments for Alzheimer's Disease (and Non-Alzheimer's Dementia)

There are at least three natural treatments for Alzheimer's disease with significant scientific evidence behind them: ginkgo, phosphatidylserine, and L-acetyl-carnitine.

Ginkgo: Strong Evidence It Improves
Memory and Mental Function

The most well-established herbal treatment for Alzheimer's disease (and, indeed, one of the few herbs that probably deserves the description "proven effective") is the ancient herb *Ginkgo biloba.* Ginkgo, the oldest surviving species of tree, has been traced back 300 million years. Although it died out in Europe during the Ice Age, ginkgo survived in

China, Japan, and other parts of East Asia. It has been cultivated extensively for both ceremonial and medical purposes, and some especially revered trees have been lovingly tended for over 1,000 years. Asian herbalists used ginkgo seeds to treat asthma and other conditions.

In Europe, researchers focused on ginkgo leaf, using standardized extracts of it rather than the whole herb. By 1995, ginkgo-leaf extract had become the most widely prescribed herb in Germany. Today, German family physicians generally favor it above all drug treatments for dementia.[1]

Ginkgo is also used to treat intermittent claudication (see the discussion of ginkgo under Intermittent Claudication), tinnitus, impotence (see Impotence), depression (see Depression), macular degeneration (see Macular Degeneration), and PMS symptoms (see PMS), although with much less evidence than for dementia. (For more information on ginkgo, see *The Natural Pharmacist Guide to Ginkgo and Memory.*)

What Is the Scientific Evidence for Ginkgo?
The scientific record for ginkgo is extensive and impressive. According to a 1992 article published in *Lancet,* over 40 double-blind controlled trials had been performed by that date, evaluating the benefits of ginkgo in treating age-related mental decline.[2] Of these studies, which involved about 1,000 participants, eight were rated of good quality and all but one produced positive results. Most of these studies were performed prior to a full recognition of the identity of Alzheimer's disease, but they are presumed to have involved both Alzheimer's and non-Alzheimer's cases. The authors of the *Lancet* article felt that the evidence was strong enough to conclude that ginkgo extract is an effective treatment for severe age-related mental decline.

Studies since 1992 have provided additional evidence for this conclusion.[3,4] Interestingly, German physicians are so certain that ginkgo is effective that they find it difficult to perform scientific studies of the herb. To them, it is unethical to give a placebo to people with Alzheimer's when they could be taking ginkgo instead and have additional months of useful life ahead.[5] This objection does not apply in the United States, where physicians do not prescribe ginkgo.

A recent study published in the *Journal of the American Medical Association* reported the results of a year-long double-blind trial of ginkgo in over 300 people with Alzheimer's or non-Alzheimer's dementia.[6] Participants were given either 40 mg of the ginkgo extract or a placebo 3 times daily. The results showed that 27% of the treated group showed significant improvement on an overall rating scale that evaluates the severity of Alzheimer's disease, compared to only 14% in the placebo group. Also, 40% of those given placebo worsened over the course of the study, whereas only 19% of the treated participants worsened.

The study authors interpret these statistics to mean that in about 20% of cases, ginkgo may slow the development of Alzheimer's disease by 6 months to 1 year. These results do not make ginkgo out to be a miracle cure, but they do confirm that it is a useful treatment for dementia.

How Does Ginkgo Work?

In the past, scientists believed that dementia was caused by a reduced blood and oxygen supply to the brain. Because ginkgo appears to improve circulation (as described under Intermittent Claudication), European physicians assumed that ginkgo was simply getting more blood to brain cells and thereby making them work better. However, advances in the understanding of age-related mental decline have led scientists to move away from this theory. Ginkgo is now believed to function by directly stimulating nerve cell activity and protecting nerve cells from further injury.[7]

Dosage

The standard dosage of ginkgo is 40 to 80 mg 3 times daily of a 50:1 extract standardized to contain 24% ginkgo-flavone glycosides.

Safety Issues

Ginkgo appears to be very safe. Extremely high doses have been given to animals for long periods of time without serious consequences.[8]

In all the clinical trials of ginkgo up to 1991, which have involved almost 10,000 people, the incidence of side effects produced by ginkgo extract was extremely small. Only 21 cases of gastrointestinal discomfort were reported, and even fewer cases of headaches, dizziness, and allergic skin reactions.[9]

However, ginkgo is known to "thin" the blood, and highly regarded journals have reported cases of bleeding in the skull and the iris chamber associated with ginkgo use.[10,11] For this reason, ginkgo should not be combined with drugs that also thin the blood, such as Coumadin (warfarin), heparin, Trental (pentoxifylline), or even aspirin. In most German studies of ginkgo, participants were not allowed to take any blood thinners. There may conceivably be risks in combining ginkgo with natural substances that thin the blood as well, such as garlic and high-dose vitamin E, although there have been no reports of such problems. Ginkgo should also be used with caution, if at all, by those with bleeding disorders such as hemophilia, or during the periods before or after surgery and prior to labor and delivery.

Safety for pregnant or nursing women and those with severe liver or kidney disease has not been established.

Phosphatidylserine: Good Evidence of Effectiveness

Like ginkgo, the supplement phosphatidylserine is widely used in Europe to treat various forms of dementia. Phosphatidylserine is one of the many substances involved in the structure and maintenance of cell membranes. While it is tempting to speculate that phosphatidylserine works by strengthening nerve cells against damage, we really don't know how this supplement works.

What Is the Scientific Evidence for Phosphatidylserine?

Phosphatidylserine appears to produce significant improvements in memory, mental function, and behavior in those with moderate to severe mental decline. The largest study of phosphatidylserine followed 494 elderly individuals in northeastern Italy over a course of 6 months.[12] The benefits produced by phosphatidylserine were roughly comparable to what has been seen with ginkgo.

Other double-blind studies performed over the last decade, involving a total of more than 500 people with age-related cognitive decline, have shown similarly positive results.[13–21]

Dosage

The standard dosage of phosphatidylserine is 100 to 200 mg 3 times daily; however, some studies have used 200 mg twice daily. After full effects are achieved, a lower dosage of 100 mg daily may be sufficient to maintain good results.

Safety Issues

Phosphatidylserine is generally regarded as safe. Side effects are rare and are typically limited to mild gastrointestinal distress. However, there are concerns that phosphatidylserine may interact with the blood-thinning drug heparin.[22] Maximum safe doses in young children, pregnant or nursing women, and those with severe liver or kidney disease has not been established.

L-Acetyl-Carnitine: May Be Slightly Helpful

Carnitine is a vitamin-like substance that is often used for congestive heart failure and other heart conditions (see the discussions of carnitine under Angina and Congestive Heart Failure). A special form of carnitine, L-acetyl-carnitine, sometimes called acetyl-L-carnitine, appears to be useful in Alzheimer's disease. Although we don't know precisely how it works, it may mimic the effects of the naturally occurring brain chemical acetylcholine, which is found in lower-than-normal levels in the brains of people with Alzheimer's disease.

What Is the Scientific Evidence for L-Acetyl-Carnitine?

Several large double-blind and single-blind studies, involving a total of more than 1,400 people, suggest that L-acetyl-carnitine may relieve symptoms and slow the progression of Alzheimer's disease and other forms of dementia.[23–33] One of these studies followed 130 people with the clinical diagnosis of Alzheimer's disease for 1 year.[34] The treated group showed a slower rate of deterioration in 13 of 14 measurements of dementia. However, one recent large study failed to find statistically significant benefit. [35] The probable explanation is that L-acetyl-carnitine is only slightly effective.

Dosage

A typical dosage of L-acetyl-carnitine is 500 to 1,000 mg 3 times daily.

Safety Issues

L-acetyl-carnitine appears to be a very safe substance.[36] However, individuals on dialysis should not receive this (or any other supplement) without a physician's supervision. The maximum safe dosage in pregnant or nursing women and those with severe liver or kidney disease has not been established.

Other Natural Treatments for Alzheimer's Disease (and Non-Alzheimer's Dementia)

Preliminary evidence suggests that vitamin E at the high dosage of 2,000 IU daily may slow the progression of

Alzheimer's disease.[37] A physician's supervision is essential when taking this much vitamin E due to risks of bleeding complications.

Vitamin C, phosphatidylcholine, zinc, magnesium, DHEA, and vitamin B_{12} have also been suggested as treatments for Alzheimer's disease. However, there has not yet been sufficient scientific investigation to confirm their effectiveness.

ANGINA

Principal Natural Treatments
L-carnitine and L-propionyl-carnitine
Other Natural Treatments
Coenzyme Q_{10}, magnesium, hawthorn, khella, *Coleus forskohlii*

Essentially, angina is a muscle cramp in the heart—the one muscle that cannot take a rest. It develops when the heart muscle does not receive enough oxygen for its needs.

People usually experience angina as a squeezing chest pain, similar to a heavy weight or a tight band, accompanied by sweating, shortness of breath, and possibly pain radiating into the left arm or neck. Usually, angina is brought on by exercise—the more rapidly the heart pumps, the more oxygen it needs. Atherosclerosis (hardening of the arteries) is the most common cause of angina.

Conventional treatment for angina is very effective. Drugs that expand (dilate) the heart's arteries, such as nitroglycerin, can give immediate relief. Other drugs help over the long term by making the heart's work easier. Surgical treatments (such as angioplasty and coronary artery bypass grafting) physically widen the blood vessels that feed the heart.

To prevent heart attacks, current recommendations suggest that most people take daily doses of aspirin, make lifestyle changes such as diet and exercise to lower cholesterol, and reduce other factors that accelerate atherosclerosis.

Principal Natural Treatments for Angina

Angina is a serious disease that absolutely requires conventional medical evaluation and supervision. No one should self-treat for angina. However, alternative treatments can provide a useful adjunct to standard medical care when monitored by an appropriate health-care professional. I intentionally do not give dosages in this section as they should be individualized by your physician.

L-Carnitine

Double-blind studies suggest that the vitamin-like substance L-carnitine can relieve angina symptoms. Carnitine plays a role in the cellular production of energy. Although carnitine does not address the cause of angina, it appears to help the heart produce energy more efficiently, thereby enabling it to get by with less oxygen.

In a double-blind study involving 200 participants, carnitine improved angina symptoms in people also taking standard medications.[1] Over the 6 months of the study, the carnitine-treated group showed significant improvement in exercise tolerance and a lower incidence of abnormal electrocardiogram readings. Side effects were negligible. A special form of carnitine, known as L-propionyl-carnitine, may be even more effective.[2] Consult with your physician regarding dosage and specific safety issues. (For more information on Carnitine, see *The Natural Pharmacist: Your Complete Guide to Vitamins and Supplements.*)

Other Natural Treatments for Angina

Coenzyme Q_{10} (CoQ_{10}) is best known as a treatment for congestive heart failure, but it may offer benefits in angina as well.[3] Magnesium has also shown some promise.[4] Although there is little direct evidence, the herbs hawthorn, khella, and *Coleus forskohlii* may also be useful.

Lifestyle Approaches

In the long term, restoring your heart's arteries back to normal is the best thing you can do for your angina. The famous Lifestyle Heart Trial, conducted by Dr. Dean Ornish, showed that people who adopt a lowfat vegetarian diet and other healthful lifestyle habits can actually reverse the level of blockage in their coronary arteries.[5]

Absolute vegetarianism is not essential for good results. In general, eating a diet low in red meat and high in whole grains and fresh fruits and vegetables seems wise. Olive oil and canola oil appear to be among the healthiest vegetable oils for use in cooking (for additional suggestions, see the discussion under Atherosclerosis).

ANXIETY AND PANIC ATTACKS

Principal Natural Treatments

Kava

Other Natural Treatments

Valerian, skullcap, hops, lemon balm, GABA, selenium, flax oil, general multivitamin

As Kierkegaard pointed out long ago, we live in the age of anxiety. Most of us suffer from chronic anxiety to some extent because modern life is jagged, fast-paced, and divorced from the natural rhythms that tend to create a harmonious inner life. The calming cycles of farming, the instinctive satisfactions of hunting and gathering, and pure faith in religion gave our ancestors inner resources that few of us possess today.

People who suffer from the emotional illness called anxiety disorder, however, go a step beyond this common feeling. The quality of their lives is significantly diminished by the pervading presence of fear, which is often unrelated to any obvious cause. Even if a cause can be identified, the magnitude of anxiety they experience is greater than the actual degree of stress.

Typical symptoms of anxiety disorder include feelings of tension, irritability, worry, frustration, turmoil, and hopelessness, along with insomnia, restless sleep, grinding of teeth, jaw pain, an inability to sit still, and an incapacity to cope. Physical sensations frequently arise as well, including a characteristic feeling of being unable to take a full, satisfying breath; dry mouth; rapid heartbeat; heart palpitations; a lump in the throat; tightness in the chest; and cramping in the bowels. Anxiety can also give rise to panic attacks. These may be so severe that they are mistaken for heart attacks. The heart pounds and palpitates, the chest feels tight and painful, and the whole body tenses with unreasoning fear. Such attacks can be triggered by anxiety-provoking situations, but they may also come out of nowhere, perhaps even awakening you from sleep. When a person tends to suffer more from panic attacks than generalized anxiety, physicians call the illness *panic disorder.*

The medical treatment of anxiety involves mainly anti-anxiety drugs. Some, such as Xanax, are effective immediately; others, such as BuSpar, take a week or more to reach full effect. Antidepressant drugs may also be helpful. Panic attacks are generally more difficult to treat than other aspects of anxiety.

Medications are best used in the short term, and it is advisable to seek more permanent help through psychotherapy.

Principal Natural Treatments for Anxiety

The herb kava is widely used in Europe as a medical treatment for anxiety.

Kava: Widely Used in Europe for Anxiety

In Europe, the herb kava is widely prescribed for anxiety. Kava is a member of the pepper family that has long been cultivated by Pacific Islanders for use as a social and ceremonial drink. The first description of kava came to the West from Captain James Cook on his celebrated voyages through the South Seas. Cook reported that when village elders and chieftains occasionally gathered for significant meetings, they would hold an elaborate kava ceremony at the beginning to break the ice. Typically, each participant would drink two or three bowls of chewed-up kava mixed with coconut milk. They also drank kava in less formal social settings as a mild intoxicant.

When European scientists learned about kava's effects, they set to work trying to isolate its active principles. However, it was not until 1966 that substances named *kavalactones* were isolated and shown to be effective on their own. One of the most active of these is the chemical dihydrokavain, which has been found to produce a sedative, painkilling, and anticonvulsant action.[1,2,3] Other named kavalactones include kavain, methysticin, and dihydromethysticin.

High doses of kava extracts cause muscular relaxation and, at very high doses, paralysis without loss of consciousness.[4–7] Kava is also a local anesthetic, producing peculiar numbing sensations when held in the mouth

Germany's Commission E, that country's official herb-regulating body, has authorized the use of kava as a medical treatment for "states of nervous anxiety, tension, and agitation." It is also used for insomnia (see the discussion of kava under Insomnia). (For more information on kava, see *The Natural Pharmacist Guide to Kava and Anxiety*.)

What Is the Scientific Evidence for Kava?

According to double-blind studies involving a total of more than 400 participants, kava appears to be an effective treatment for symptoms of anxiety. The best study was a 6-month double-blind trial that tested kava's effectiveness in 100 individuals with various forms of anxiety.[8] Over the course of the trial, they were evaluated with a list of questions called the Hamilton Anxiety Scale (HAM-A). The HAM-A assigns a total score based on symptoms such as restlessness, nervousness, heart palpitations, stomach discomfort, dizziness, and chest pain. Lower scores indicate reduced anxiety.

Although it took a while for results to develop, by 8 weeks participants who were given kava showed significantly improved HAM-A scores compared to the placebo group. These good results were sustained throughout the duration of the treatment. Interestingly, previous studies had showed a good response in 1 week, especially in menopause-related anxiety.[9,10,11] How fast does kava really work? We will need additional research to know for sure, but you should probably give it a couple of months before deciding whether it works for you.

Another study compared kava against standard antianxiety drugs. For a period of 6 weeks, 174 people with symptoms of anxiety were given either kava or one of two antianxiety medications (oxazepam and bromazepam).[12] Improvement in HAM-A scores was about the same in both groups. However, for technical reasons this study didn't actually prove that kava is equally effective as those standard medications.

Although we don't know exactly how kava functions in the body, its method of action seems to involve brain receptors for a substance known as gamma–aminobutyric acid (GABA).[13] This would make it similar to benzodiazepine drugs like Valium and Xanax. GABA is believed to

play a role in anxiety that is somewhat similar to serotonin's role in depression, although there are many gaps in
our knowledge.

Dosage

Kava is usually sold in a standardized form for which the
total dose of kavalactones per pill is listed. The dose used
should supply about 40 to 70 mg of kavalactones 3 times
daily. The total daily dosage should not exceed 300 mg of
kavalactones. Be patient, because the benefits may take a
while to develop (see What Is the Scientific Evidence for
Kava?).

Safety Issues

When taken appropriately, kava appears to be quite safe.
Animal studies have shown that doses up to 4 times the
normal dose cause no harm at all, and 13 times the normal
dose causes only mild problems in rats.[14]

A study of 4,049 participants who took a rather low dose
of kava (70 mg of kavalactones daily) for 7 weeks found side
effects in 1.5% of cases.[15] These were mostly mild gastrointestinal complaints and allergic rashes. A 4-week study of
3,029 people, who were given a more realistic 240 mg of
kavalactones daily, showed a 2.3% incidence of basically the
same side effects.[16]

However, long-term use (months to years) of kava in excess of 400 mg kavalactones daily can create a very distinc-
tive dry, scaly rash called "kava dermopathy."[17] It disappears
promptly when the kava use stops.

Studies suggest that kava does not produce mental
cloudiness or impair driving ability when used at normal
doses,[18–21] however I still would not recommend driving
while taking it.

European physicians have not reported any problems
with kava addiction.[22] However, one study in mice suggests that addiction might be possible.[23]

Because high doses of kava can cause inebriation, concern exists that it could become an herb of abuse. There have been reports of young people trying to get high by taking products that they thought contained kava. As it turned out, one of these products, fX, turned out to contain dangerous drugs but no kava at all.

Kava should not be combined with alcohol, prescription antianxiety drugs, sedatives, or other drugs that depress mental function. Reports suggest that the combination of kava and benzodiazepine drugs (in the Valium family) can lead to coma.[24]

Germany's Commission E warns against the use of kava during pregnancy and nursing. Safety in young children and those with severe liver or kidney disease has also not been established.

Transition from Medications to Kava

If you are taking Xanax or other drugs in the benzodiazepine family, switching to kava will be very difficult. You definitely must seek medical supervision because withdrawal symptoms can be severe and even life-threatening. Additionally, if you are taking Xanax on an "as needed" basis to stop acute panic attacks, kava cannot be expected to have the same rapidity of action.

It is easier to make the switch from milder antianxiety drugs, such as BuSpar and antidepressants. Nonetheless, a physician's supervision is still strongly advised.

Other Natural Treatments for Anxiety

The following natural treatments are widely recommended for anxiety, but they have not been scientifically proven effective at this time.

Valerian: May Provide Calming Effects

The herb valerian is best known as a remedy for insomnia. However, according to one preliminary double-blind study, it also produces calming effects in stressful situations.[25] The standard dosage is 2 to 3 g twice daily.

Valerian is generally regarded as safe. However, safety in young children, pregnant or nursing women, and those with severe liver or kidney disease has not been established. At press time, there has been an unconfirmed report of severe withdrawal symptoms after extended use of valerian. (For other comments regarding dosage and safety, see the discussion of valerian under Insomnia.)

Other Herbs
Other herbs that are frequently recommended for anxiety include skullcap, hops, and lemon balm.

GABA: No Evidence That It Is Effective
Because GABA (gamma–aminobutyric acid) is known to play a central role in anxiety, some alternative practitioners suggest simply taking this amino acid as a supplement. However, no scientific evidence suggests that orally ingested GABA gets to where it can do any good.

Other Supplements
Supplementation with selenium (200 mcg daily), flax oil (2 to 6 tablespoons daily), or a general multivitamin are all said to help relieve anxiety symptoms in some people.

ASTHMA

Principal Natural Treatments
Tylophora, *Coleus forskohlii,* vitamin C, ma huang (unsafe)
Other Natural Treatments
Vitamin B_{12}, quercetin, vitamin B_6, antioxidants, essential fatty acids, magnesium, licorice, grindelia, garlic, onions, marshmallow, mullein, *Lobelia inflata*

People who are having an asthma attack have real trouble taking a breath. Many people with stuffy noses from hay fever or colds say, "I can't breathe," but they retain the option of breathing through the mouth. Asthmatics, however, know what "I can't breathe" really means. Instead of their nasal passages, it is the bronchial tubes in their lungs that become swollen and clogged. Breathing can become frighteningly difficult.

Asthma involves two conditions: (1) contraction of the small muscles surrounding the bronchial tubes and (2) swelling of the lining of those tubes. Until recently, treatment usually addressed the first aspect of asthma; but in the last decade, it has become clear that tissue swelling is more fundamental.

Conventional medical treatment for asthma involves bronchodilators, which relax the bronchial muscles, and anti-inflammatory medication, which helps relieve the swelling of tissue. The most effective treatments for reducing this inflammation are steroids, inhalable forms of which have been developed that do not cause as many side effects as oral drugs, such as prednisone. Nonsteroidal drugs, such as cromolyn (Intal), are also available.

The conventional treatment of asthma is highly effective in most cases.

Principal Natural Treatments for Asthma

Perhaps the most promising natural treatment for asthma is the herb tylophora. Another herb, *Coleus forskohlii,* may also be helpful, but it is really more like a drug than an herb. Vitamin C also appears to be somewhat helpful. The Chinese herb ma huang is definitely effective for mild asthma, but it isn't safe.

Tylophora: A Promising Treatment for Asthma

The herb *Tylophora indica* (also called *Tylophora asthmatica*), appears to offer considerable promise as a treatment for asthma. It has a long history of use in the traditional Ayurvedic medicine of India. In a small 4-week, double-blind study, individuals who were given 40 mg of a tylophora alcohol extract daily for 6 days showed significant improvement, and this improvement only gradually faded away after use of the herb was stopped.[1] Other studies have shown similar results.[2,3] However, these studies are 20 years old or more, and they were not conducted according to modern scientific standards. Larger and better studies are necessary to discover whether tylophora is truly effective.

The typical dosage of tylophora leaf is 200 mg twice daily. Its safety has not been fully evaluated, and for this reason it should not be used by children, pregnant or nursing women, or those with severe kidney or liver disease. Whether tylophora interacts with any drugs is unknown. Tylophora occasionally causes mild digestive distress, mouth soreness, and altered taste sensation.

Coleus forskohlii: *May Be Effective, but More Like a Drug Than an Herb*

Another herb often recommended for asthma also comes from India, *Coleus forskohlii*. However, I cannot give it a wholehearted recommendation. *Coleus forskohlii* contains a powerful substance called forskolin, which produces far-reaching effects in the body, perhaps relieving asthma symptoms. Unfortunately, we do not know the implications of all its other effects.

Natural *Coleus forskohlii* contains only small amounts of forskolin. However, manufacturers deliberately modify the herb to dramatically increase its forskolin content, making it more like a drug than an herb. Forskolin appears to be safe, but more studies need to be undertaken before it can be recommended for self-treatment.

Vitamin C: Appears to Provide Some Benefits

Many studies have been conducted on the effects of vitamin C in treating asthma. When you put all the results together, it appears that the regular use of high-dose vitamin C provides some benefits.[4,5] A typical dosage is 1 to 3 g daily.

Vitamin C at this dosage has not been definitely associated with any significant harm. However, because high dose of vitamin C can cause copper deficiency, you should also take 1 to 3 mg of copper daily. Diarrhea is a common side effect, but it usually goes away in a week or so. There is no direct evidence that vitamin C poses a risk for people with a history of kidney stones, but caution is recommended.

Ma Huang: Effective, but Not Safe

The Chinese herb ma huang is definitely effective for mild asthma, because it contains the drug ephedrine. However, I cannot recommend using it because of safety concerns. This Chinese herb is a member of a primitive family of plants that look like thin, branching, connected straws. A related species, *Ephedra nevadensis*, grows wild in the American Southwest and is widely called Mormon tea. However, only the Asian species of ephedra contains the active compounds ephedrine and pseudoephedrine.

Ma huang was traditionally used by Chinese herbalists in the early stages of respiratory infections and for the short-term treatment of certain kinds of asthma, eczema, hay fever, narcolepsy, and edema. However, ma huang was not supposed to be taken for an extended period of time, and people with less than robust constitutions were warned to use only low doses or to avoid ma huang altogether.

Japanese chemists isolated ephedrine from ma huang at the turn of the twentieth century, and it soon became a primary treatment for asthma in the United States and abroad. Ephedra's other major ingredient, pseudoephedrine, became the decongestant Sudafed.

Although ephedrine can still be found in a few over-the-counter asthma drugs, physicians seldom prescribe it today. The problem is that ephedrine mimics the effects of adrenaline and causes symptoms such as rapid heart-beat, high blood pressure, agitation, insomnia, nausea, and loss of appetite. The newer asthma drugs are much safer and easier to tolerate. This is a situation in which synthetic drugs are less dangerous than a natural one. I do not recommend using ma huang for asthma.

Other Natural Treatments for Asthma

The following natural treatments for asthma are often widely recommended, but they have not been scientifically proven effective at this time.

Vitamin B_{12}

Supplementation with vitamin B_{12} is said to be effective for asthma.[6] However, the scientific evidence in its favor consists almost entirely of open studies that did not attempt to eliminate the placebo effect.

Quercetin

The flavonoid quercetin is often recommended as a treatment for asthma on the basis of test-tube studies that show that it can inhibit the release of inflammatory substances from special cells called mast cells. Because the asthma drugs Intal and Tilade are believed to work in the same way, many natural medicine authorities have often recommended quercetin as an equivalent treatment. However, even though significant direct evidence exists that Tilade and Intal actually work, no such evidence yet exists for quercetin. Interestingly, Intal is derived from a Mediterranean herb named khella.

Vitamin B₆

Vitamin B_6 is often mentioned as a treatment for asthma, but the evidence that it works is weak and contradictory. A double-blind study of 76 asthmatic children found significant benefit after 1 month.[7] Children in the treated group were able to reduce their doses of bronchodilators and steroids. However, a recent double-blind study of 31 adults who also used either inhaled or oral steroids did not show any benefit.[8]

The dosages of vitamin B_6 used in these studies were quite high, in the range of 200 to 300 mg daily. Because of the risk of nerve injury, it is not advisable to take this much without medical supervision.

Antioxidants

Antioxidants, such as vitamin E, beta-carotene, and selenium, are frequently recommended for asthma on the grounds that they may protect inflamed lung tissue. However, there is little direct scientific evidence that they work at this time.

Essential Fatty Acids

The essential fatty acids in fish oil, flax oil, and evening primrose oil are suspected to inhibit inflammatory responses such as those that occur in asthma. However, most of the studies that tried fish oil as a treatment for asthma came up with negative results.[9–16]

Magnesium

Magnesium is frequently mentioned as a treatment for asthma, but no good studies have shown that oral magnesium is helpful. Some evidence exists that intravenous and inhaled magnesium may offer some short-term benefit,[17,18] but the relevance of these findings to taking magnesium supplements by mouth is unclear.

Other Herbs

Other traditional asthma treatments include the herbs licorice, grindelia, garlic, onions, marshmallow, and mullein. *Lobelia inflata* is a traditional herbal treatment for asthma; but according to traditional directions, it should be taken to the point of vomiting, a process I can hardly recommend.

ATHEROSCLEROSIS
(Prevention)

Principal Natural Treatments

Antioxidant supplements: vitamin E, vitamin C (in combination with vitamin E or alone), garlic, selenium, proanthocyanidins (PCOs) from grape seed or pine bark, lipoic acid, turmeric, resveratrol, coenzyme Q_{10}

Other Natural Treatments

Essential fatty acids, aortic glycosaminoglycans, bilberry, ginger, ginkgo, feverfew, dong quai, hawthorn, lifestyle changes

Not Recommended Treatments

Beta-carotene

Atherosclerosis, or hardening of the arteries, is the leading cause of death in men over age 35 and all people over 45. Most heart attacks and strokes are due to atherosclerosis. Although the origin of this condition is not completely understood, we know that it is accelerated by factors such as high blood pressure, high cholesterol, diabetes, smoking, and physical inactivity.

Current theories suggest that atherosclerosis begins with injury to the lining of arteries. High blood pressure physically stresses this lining, while circulating substances such as low-density lipoprotein (LDL) cholesterol, homocysteine, free radicals, and nicotine chemically damage it. White blood cells then attach to the damaged wall and take up residence. Then, for reasons that are not entirely clear, they begin to accumulate cholesterol and other fats. Platelets also latch on, releasing substances that cause the formation of fibrous tissue. The overall effect is a thickening of the artery wall called a fibrous plaque.

Over time, the thickening increases, narrowing the bore of the artery. When blockage reaches 75 to 90%, the person begins to notice anginal heart pains (see the discussion under Angina). In the lower legs, blockage of the blood flow leads to leg pain during exercise (see the discussion under Intermittent Claudication).

Blood clots can develop on the irregular surfaces of the artery and may become detached and block downstream blood flow. Fragments of plaque can also detach. Heart attacks are generally caused by such blood clots, whereas strokes are more often caused by plaque fragments or gradual obstruction. Furthermore, atherosclerotic blood vessels are weak and can burst.

With a disease as serious and progressive as atherosclerosis, the best treatment is prevention. Conventional medical approaches focus on lifestyle changes, such as increasing aerobic exercise, reducing the consumption of saturated fats, and quitting smoking. The regular use of aspirin also appears to be quite helpful by preventing platelet attachment and blood clot formation. If necessary, drugs may be used to lower cholesterol levels or blood pressure.

Recently, conventional medicine has also begun to suggest keeping levels of homocysteine low by adding supplemental folic acid and vitamin B_6 to the diet. Consult with your physician for late-breaking information regarding the ideal dose of these supplements. At the time of this writing, recommendations suggest 400 to 800 mcg of folic acid daily along with 10 to 20 mg of vitamin B_6.

Because the following material is so complex, I have summarized this information in the section called Putting It All Together. You can skip to it now if you want just the conclusions.

Principal Natural Treatments for Preventing Atherosclerosis

In the field of preventing atherosclerosis, conventional and alternative approaches overlap. Natural medicine supports (indeed, it first championed) many of the lifestyle changes now encouraged by conventional medicine. Many other "alternative" treatments are on the verge of acceptance into conventional medicine.

Many studies have been performed to determine precisely which nutrients are most helpful in preventing atherosclerosis. However, it is tricky to interpret the results of this research.

The most common and potentially most confusing type of study is the *observational study*. This study follows large groups of people for years and keeps track of a great deal of information about them, including diet. Researchers then examine the data closely and try to identify which dietary factors are associated with better health and longer life.

However, the results can be misleading. For example, if an observational study finds that people who take vitamin supplements live longer, it is not necessarily the vitamins that deserve the credit. Vitamin users also tend to exercise more and to eat more healthful foods, habits that may play a more important role than the vitamins. It is hard to tell.

A more reliable kind of study is the *intervention trial*. In these studies, some people are given a certain vitamin and then compared to others who are given a placebo (or sometimes no treatment at all). The best intervention trials use a double-blind design. The results of intervention trials are far more conclusive than those of observational studies. Unfortunately, they are very expensive to perform, and relatively few have been completed.

This section details the evidence that is available to date. Because this is such a rapidly changing field, new evidence will likely have been found by the time you read this book. Consult a health-care professional for the latest information.

(For natural treatments that may reduce two important risk factors for atherosclerosis, see the discussions under Cholesterol and Hypertension.)

Antioxidants: Increasingly
Accepted by Conventional Medicine

The body is engaged in a constant battle against damaging chemicals called *free radicals*, or pro-oxidants. These highly reactive substances are believed to play a major role in atherosclerosis, cancer, and aging in general.

To counter the harmful effects of free radicals, the body manufactures antioxidants to chemically neutralize them. However, the natural antioxidant system may not always be equal to the task. Sources of free radicals, such as cigarette smoke and smoked meat, may overwhelm this defense mechanism. In the not-too-distant future, tests of "antioxidant status" may join cholesterol and blood pressure as standard components of preventive medicine screening.

Certain dietary nutrients augment the body's natural antioxidants and may be able to help out when the primary system is under stress. Vitamins E and C and beta-carotene are the best known, but many other substances found in fruits and vegetables are also strong antioxidants.

It appears that antioxidants can help prevent atherosclerosis. However, precisely which ones are most effective remains an area of active study.

Vitamin E: Dramatically Reduces Heart Attacks

Vitamin E is the best-documented antioxidant supplement for the prevention of heart disease. Most of the evidence comes from observational studies, but a few intervention trials have shown this as well.

In a double-blind intervention trial of 2,002 people with proven coronary artery disease, 546 were given 800 IU of vitamin E daily, 489 were given 400 IU daily, and 967 were given placebo.[1] Participants were followed for an average of about 18 months. The treated individuals showed an almost 80% drop in nonfatal heart attacks. Curiously, fatal heart attacks were not reduced, for reasons that are unclear.

However, two other very large intervention trials (1,862 and 29,133 participants, respectively) found no benefit.[2,3] These trials involved smokers who were given only 50 IU of vitamin E daily. It may be that vitamin E, especially at this relatively low dosage, cannot counter the powerful negative influence of smoking.

Observational studies have also given a strong indication that vitamin E can help prevent atherosclerosis. In one study of 11,178 people aged 67 to 105 years, those participants who were taking vitamin E supplements at the beginning of the study were found to have a 34% reduced likelihood of death from heart disease.[4] Vitamin C supplements alone did not seem to make a difference, but the combination of vitamin E and C produced a 53% reduction in risk. Long-term use of vitamin E appeared to be associated with an even greater risk reduction of 63%.

It makes sense that the combination of vitamin C and E would be especially beneficial because vitamin E fights free radicals that dissolve in fats while vitamin C fights those that dissolve in water. Together, the coverage would be expected to be very complete.

In another large observational study, 39,910 U.S. male health professionals were followed for 4 years.[5] Vitamin E supplementation of 100 IU or more daily was associated with a 37% reduced risk of heart disease.

Vitamin E seems to be helpful for women, too. An 8-year study of 87,245 female nurses aged 34 to 59 with no previously diagnosed heart disease found that women who took vitamin E supplements for at least 2 years had a 40% reduced risk of developing coronary disease.[6] Consumption of other antioxidants was not associated with much risk reduction.

Keep in mind, however, that observational studies are not completely reliable. As described previously, people who take supplements also tend to have healthier lifestyle habits, which makes it difficult to interpret the results. We need more, better intervention trials to know for sure.

It is not clear how vitamin E works. One theory points out that vitamin E protects fats and cholesterol from being converted by free radicals into unhealthy chemicals.[7] However, an animal study casts doubt on whether this is really significant.[8] Another possible explanation points to vitamin E's effects on the formation of dangerous blood clots. Like aspirin, which is known to help prevent heart attacks, vitamin E interferes with the activity of platelets.[9] As mentioned earlier, platelets stick to the walls of blood vessels that have been damaged by atherosclerosis, forming blood clots that can then break off and cause obstructions downstream. Aspirin is believed to help prevent heart attacks and strokes by interfering with blood clots, and vitamin E may do the same.

The optimum dose of vitamin E is not known. A typical recommendation is 400 IU daily. This dosage is generally believed to be safe. However, in one study, vitamin E supplementation was associated with an increase in hemorrhagic stroke, the kind of stroke caused by bleeding.[10] This is not completely surprising considering vitamin E's ability to reduce blood clotting.[11] Certainly, vitamin E should not be combined with aspirin or prescription blood thinners except under a physician's supervision. On the other hand, some evidence exists that combination treatment with vitamin E and aspirin may offer additional benefits in preventing the more common kind of stroke caused by obstruction, so you may want to discuss this whole subject with your physician.[12] I definitely do not recommend taking more than 800 IU daily except on medical advice.

Vitamin C: Best with Vitamin E

As noted earlier, vitamin C may offer added benefit when it is combined with vitamin E. However the evidence that vitamin C supplements taken by themselves are helpful for atherosclerosis is weak.[13,14,15] There have been about as many positive as negative studies. Foods containing vitamin C do appear to be helpful, probably because they contain numerous other healthy substances as well.

Beta-Carotene: Best in Food, Not As a Supplement

The study results involving beta-carotene are interesting. Beta-carotene is one member of a large category of substances found in foods known as *carotenes*, which are found in high levels in yellow, orange, and dark-green vegetables.

Many studies suggest that eating foods high in carotenes can prevent atherosclerosis.[16] However, isolated beta-carotene in supplement form may not help, and could actually increase your risk.

A huge double-blind intervention trial involving 29,133 Finnish male smokers found 11% *more* deaths from heart disease and 15 to 20% *more* strokes in those participants taking beta-carotene supplements.[17] This study was mentioned in the vitamin E section previously. Vitamin E was not found to be helpful, but at least it did not cause harm. Beta-carotene actually increased deaths from heart attacks and strokes. This certainly does not encourage one to take it.

Similar poor results with beta-carotene were seen in another large double-blind study in smokers.[18] Furthermore, beta-carotene supplementation was also found to increase the incidence of angina in smokers.[19]

What is happening here? Clearly, smoking presents a challenge to antioxidants. Vitamin E, so protective in other circumstances, seems to have a difficult time protecting smokers. However, the question remains: Why should beta-carotene not only fail to help but actually worsen the situation?

One possible explanation is that beta-carotene in the diet always comes along with other naturally occurring carotenes. It is quite likely that other carotenoids in the diet are equally or more important than beta-carotene alone.[20] Taking beta-carotene supplements may actually promote deficiencies of other natural carotenes,[21] and overall that may hurt more than it helps.

The moral of the story is that you should eat your vegetables but maybe not take beta-carotene supplements.

Garlic: Lowers Cholesterol and May Provide Other Benefits

There is strong evidence that garlic can lower cholesterol (see the discussion of garlic under Cholesterol), and some evidence indicates that it can lower blood pressure as well (see the discussion of garlic under Hypertension). These two factors strongly suggest that garlic can reduce the risk of atherosclerosis. A few studies suggest that garlic can slow the development of atherosclerosis by other means as well. Garlic is a strong antioxidant, and this may explain some of its benefits.

Garlic preparations have been shown to slow the development of atherosclerosis in rats, rabbits, and human blood vessels, reducing the size of plaque deposits by nearly 50%.[22,23]

A recent observational study of 200 men and women suggests that garlic can do the same in humans as well.[24] Those who were taking 300 mg or more of garlic daily for 2 years showed a distinct improvement in the flexibility of the aorta, the main artery exiting the heart. This suggests a reduced level of atherosclerosis.

Significantly, there was no difference in cholesterol levels or blood pressure between those who regularly consumed garlic and those who did not. Therefore, it appears that garlic may also reduce atherosclerosis by other means besides affecting these two important risk factors.

Because garlic produces a blood-thinning effect, it should not be taken by those on blood thinners such as Coumadin (warfarin), heparin, Trental (pentoxifylline) and perhaps even aspirin except under medical supervision. Garlic might also conceivably cause bleeding problems if combined with other natural substances that mildly thin the blood, such as gingko and high-dose vitamin E. Do not take garlic supplements immediately prior to or after surgery, or before labor and delivery. (For more information on garlic, see *The Natural Pharmacist Guide to Garlic and Cholesterol.*)

Other Antioxidants: May Be Helpful, but Little Direct Evidence

Many other antioxidant vitamins, supplements, and herbs have been suggested as preventive treatments for atherosclerosis. Selenium, proanthocyanidins (PCOs) from grape seed or pine bark, lipoic acid, turmeric, resveratrol from red wine and grape skins, and coenzyme Q_{10} are commonly mentioned. However, although a number of interesting studies have suggested that these substances may be beneficial, the state of the evidence is still too preliminary to draw any conclusions.

Other Natural Treatments for Preventing Atherosclerosis

Although the following treatments are widely recommended for atherosclerosis, they cannot be considered scientifically proven at this time.

Essential Fatty Acids

It has been suggested that omega-3 fatty acids, such as those found in fish oil, can prevent atherosclerosis.[25] However, the overall effects of omega-3 fatty acids are complex and include both positive and negative influences. They appear to significantly decrease serum triglycerides (a good effect), leave total cholesterol alone (neutral), modestly raise LDL cholesterol (a bad effect), and even more modestly raise high-density lipoprotein, or HDL cholesterol (a good effect).[26] Fish oil may also lower blood pressure, help prevent blood clots, and lower homocysteine levels.[27] However, the net effect regarding atherosclerosis is unclear.[28,29]

Even if its benefit is unproven, fish oil does appear to be safe. Contrary to some reports, it does not seem to increase bleeding or affect blood sugar control in people with diabetes.[30]

Flax oil has been suggested as an alternative to fish oil.[31] However, it doesn't lower triglycerides, which appears to be the primary benefit of fish oil.

Aortic Glycosaminoglycans

Aortic glycosaminoglycans (GAGs) are substances obtained from the inside lining of the arteries of cows.

According to a recent double-blind study, 200 mg per day of GAGs can significantly slow the rate of thickening of arteries.[32] After 18 months of treatment, the additional layering of the inside vessel lining was 7.5 times less in the group receiving GAGs than in the placebo group. Preliminary evidence suggests that it may work in several ways: supplying material for repair of arteries, "thinning" the blood, and improving cholesterol levels.[33,34]

A typical dosage is 50 to 100 mg twice a day. Glycosaminoglycans are regarded as safe because they commonly occur in foods, although extensive safety studies have not been performed.

Other Herbs

Many herbs appear to decrease platelet stickiness—including bilberry, ginger, ginkgo, feverfew, dong quai, and hawthorn. Whether this translates into an actual benefit for preventing atherosclerosis remains unknown. (For other natural substances that may lower cholesterol or blood pressure, see the discussions under Cholesterol and Hypertension.)

Lifestyle Approaches

This fact cannot be emphasized enough: The most important way to prevent atherosclerosis involves lifestyle changes such as quitting smoking, increasing exercise, and adopting a diet high in whole grains, fruits, and vegetables and low in animal products. Olive oil and canola oil are probably among the most healthful of vegetable oils. Heating oils to high temperatures (as in fried foods) can oxidize them and make them less healthful.[35]

It has been suggested that a high level of fish in the diet protects against atherosclerosis. However, doubt has been cast on this idea.[36] Strangely, like beta-carotene, fish appears to be connected with a higher incidence of heart disease in smokers.[37]

However, this subject is very tricky to study. The possible connection between fish and heart disease was so well publicized for a while that people with the worst heart health may have started eating fish on purpose. This may have led to a situation in which the sickest people were eating fish while healthy people were not, completely muddying the results of the studies! Much more remains to be learned on this subject.

The moderate use of alcohol, and specifically red wine, appears to help prevent atherosclerosis, although this is controversial as well.[38–41] Coffee may slightly increase cardiovascular risk,[42] although some studies have shown no effect when other factors, such as smoking and diets high in animal fats (often associated with coffee use), are taken into account.[43] It has been suggested that coffee may raise homocysteine levels.[44] Coffee probably does not have a significant effect on cholesterol levels, although this is debatable as well (see also the discussion under Cholesterol).

Putting It All Together

This section is so complicated that I'd like to summarize all the information here in one place.

Little doubt exists that regular exercise and a diet high in fresh fruits and vegetables and low in animal fats can help prevent atherosclerosis. Unheated olive oil and canola oil are probably among the most healthful sources of dietary fat.

Supplemental vitamin E at a dosage around 400 IU daily probably also helps prevent atherosclerosis, and adding vitamin C should provide additional benefit.

Supplemental vitamin B_6 (10 to 20 mg daily) and folic acid (400 to 800 mcg daily) are probably also helpful because of their effects on homocysteine levels. Garlic, too, appears to be beneficial. The evidence for other herbs and supplements is promising but incomplete at present.

Finally, do not forget to take care of your cholesterol and blood pressure. (For more information, see Cholesterol and Hypertension.)

ATTENTION DEFICIT DISORDER

Principal Natural Treatments

There are no well-established natural treatments for ADD.

Other Natural Treatments

Calcium, zinc, magnesium, B vitamins, iron, trace minerals, blue-green algae, GABA, glycine, taurine, L-glutamine, L-tyrosine, St. John's wort

Originally, the term *attention deficit disorder* (ADD) referred to children who seemed incapable of concentrating at school. Today, however, the definition has broadened to include many adults as well. Characteristics of ADD include difficulty sustaining attention or completing tasks, easy distractibility, impulsive behavior, and hyperactivity (excessive movement and an inability to sit still). These problems make it difficult to succeed at work or at school.

Conventional treatment focuses on stimulants such as caffeine, Dexedrine, and Ritalin. These drugs produce a paradoxically calming effect in people with ADD, for reasons we don't understand. Certain antidepressants may also be useful.

Natural Treatments for Attention Deficit Disorder

There are no well-documented alternative treatments for ADD. Two authors sympathetic to natural medicine reviewed all the literature in print on a few widely recommended options: supplementation with niacin, vitamin B_6, and multivitamin and mineral tablets.[1] They failed to find any evidence of a positive effect. Nonetheless, there are some supplements that alternative practitioners feel may be effective. These include calcium, zinc, magnesium, B vitamins, iron, trace minerals, blue-green algae, and the amino acids GABA, glycine, taurine, L-glutamine, and L-tyrosine. St. John's wort is also sometimes recommended.

BENIGN PROSTATIC HYPERPLASIA
(Prostate Enlargement)

Principal Natural Treatments
Saw palmetto, pygeum, nettle root, beta-sitosterol, grass pollen
Other Natural Treatments
Pumpkin seeds, zinc, flax oil

If you're a man, and you live long enough, you will almost certainly develop benign prostatic hyperplasia (BPH). Ninety percent of all men show signs of such prostatic enlargement by the age of 80. Symptoms include difficulty in starting urination, a diminished force of urinary stream, a sensation of fullness in the bladder after urination, and the need to urinate many times at night. Ultimately, the obstruction can become so severe that urination is impossible.

The most common treatment for BPH is surgery that removes most of the prostate gland. Although this surgery is fairly safe, it is traumatic. The drugs Cardura, Flomax, Hytrin, and Proscar can relieve symptoms of BPH. In addition, Proscar has been shown to shrink the prostate and cut by half the need for surgery.

Principal Natural Treatments
for Benign Prostatic Hyperplasia

Men who suspect they may suffer from BPH should make sure to see a physician to rule out prostate cancer. After this has been done, many natural options are available that have good scientific backing. Indeed, it's hard to think of another condition for which so many natural therapies have been shown effective. (For more information on BPH, see *The Natural Pharmacist Guide to Saw Palmetto and the Prostate.*)

Saw Palmetto: A Well-Documented
Alternative to Prostate Medications

The best-documented herbal treatment for BPH is the oil of the berry of the saw palmetto tree. Saw palmetto is a native of North America; although Europeans are the principal consumers of saw palmetto, it is still grown mainly in North America.

Historically, Native Americans used saw palmetto berries for the treatment of various urinary problems in men and for breast disorders in women. European and U.S. physicians took up saw palmetto as a treatment for BPH, but in the United States the herb ultimately fell out of favor.

European interest endured, and in the 1960s French researchers discovered that, by concentrating the oils of the saw palmetto berry, they could maximize the herb's effectiveness. Subsequently, a standardized version of saw palmetto oil became an accepted treatment for prostate enlargement in New Zealand, France, Germany, Austria, Italy, Spain, and other European countries.

This herb is so well accepted in Europe that conventional drugs are considered alternative therapy for BPH! In Germany, saw palmetto is the seventh most common single-herb product prescribed. Studies suggest that benefits will develop after about 4 to 6 weeks of treatment in two-thirds of men who try it.

Saw palmetto offers two potential advantages over conventional drug treatment. The most obvious is that it usually causes no side effects. Another advantage is that saw palmetto does not change protein-specific antigen (PSA) levels. Lab tests that measure PSA are used to screen for prostate cancer. However, the widely used drug Proscar can artificially lower PSA levels, which may have the unintended effect of masking prostate cancer.

Saw palmetto is also sometimes used for chronic prostatitis. However, there is no scientific evidence that it works for this problem.

What Is the Scientific Evidence for Saw Palmetto?

The scientific evidence for saw palmetto in prostate enlargement is quite impressive.

At least seven double-blind studies involving a total of about 500 participants have compared the benefits of saw palmetto against placebo over a period of 1 to 3 months.[1–7] In all but one of these studies, the herb significantly improved urinary flow rate and most other measures of prostate disease.

A recent double-blind study followed 1,098 men who received either saw palmetto or the drug Proscar over a period of 6 months.[8] According to the results, the two treatments were about equally successful at reducing symptoms, and neither produced much in the way of side effects. However, Proscar lowered PSA levels, presenting a risk of masking prostate cancer (see the previous discussion under Saw Palmetto). Saw palmetto did not cause this problem. On the other hand, Proscar caused men's prostates to shrink by 18%, while saw palmetto only caused a 6% decrease in size, a potential advantage for the drug.

Although there are many theories about how saw palmetto works, none have been conclusively established.

The best evidence suggests that the herb interferes with male hormones.

Dosage

The standard dosage of saw palmetto is 160 mg twice daily of an extract standardized to contain 85 to 95% fatty acids and sterols. It can also be taken in one daily dose of 320 mg.[9] Taking more than this dose will not give you better results.

Note: Make sure to get a full medical checkup to rule out prostate cancer before you self-treat with saw palmetto. Furthermore, all men over the age of 50 should also continue regular prostate checkups with their physicians.

Safety Issues

Saw palmetto appears to be essentially nontoxic.[10] It's also nearly side-effect free. In a 3-year study involving 435 participants, only 34 complained of side effects, which were mainly the usual mild gastrointestinal distress.[11] No drug interactions are known.

Safety in pregnancy and nursing has not been established. However, because saw palmetto is intended for men only, this is not a terrible drawback. Those with severe liver or kidney disease should not use saw palmetto (or any other herb) except on the advice of a physician.

Pygeum: Another Well-Documented Natural Choice

The pygeum tree is a tall evergreen native to central and southern Africa. Its bark has been used since ancient times for urinary problems. In recent years, pygeum has become a popular European treatment for BPH. It's more widely used in France and Italy than in Germany. However, a comparison study with saw palmetto found that pygeum was not as effective.[12] Pygeum is also more expensive and difficult to grow.

Pygeum is also sometimes used for prostatitis, although there is as yet no significant evidence that it works.

What Is the Scientific Evidence for Pygeum?

At least 12 double-blind trials of pygeum have been performed, involving a total of over 600 participants and ranging in length from 45 to 90 days.[13] Overall, the results make a reasonably strong case that pygeum can reduce symptoms such as nighttime urination, urinary frequency, and residual urine volume. We don't know whether pygeum can reduce the need for prostate surgery, nor whether it affects PSA levels.

Dosage

The proper dosage of pygeum is 50 to 100 mg twice daily of an extract standardized to contain 14% triterpenes and 0.5% n-docosanol. It is often sold at a slightly lower dose in combination with saw palmetto.

Safety Issues

Pygeum appears to be essentially nontoxic, both in the short and the long term.[14] The most common side effect is mild gastrointestinal distress. However, safety in those with severe liver or kidney disease has not been established.

Nettle Root

Anyone who lives in a locale where nettle grows wild will likely discover the powers of this dark green plant. Depending on the species, the fine hairs on its leaves and stem cause burning pain that lasts from hours to weeks. Both its leaves and roots can be used as medicine. The root is a popular European treatment for BPH. Over a period of several months, nettle appears to reduce obstruction of urinary flow and decrease the need for nighttime urination.

Nettle leaf (not the root) is sometimes used for allergies (see the discussion of nettle leaf under Allergies).

What Is the Scientific Evidence for Nettle Root?

Nettle root has not been as well studied as saw palmetto or pygeum.

In a 4- to 6-week double-blind study of 67 men, treatment with nettle root produced a 14% improvement in urine flow and a 53% decrease in residual urine (urine that was not completely expelled from the bladder).[15] Another double-blind study of 40 men showed a significant decrease in frequency of urination after 6 months.[16] A double-blind study of 50 men over 9 weeks showed a significant improvement in urination volume.[17]

Dosage

According to Germany's Commission E, the proper dosage of nettle root is 4 to 6 g daily of the whole root or a proportional dose of concentrated extract.

Safety Issues

Nettle root appears to be nearly side-effect free. In one study of 4,087 people who took 600 to 1,200 mg of nettle daily for 6 months, less than 1% reported mild gastrointestinal distress, and only 0.19% experienced allergic reactions (skin rash).[18]

Although detailed safety studies have not been reported, no serious adverse effects have been noted in Germany, where nettle root is widely used. For theoretical reasons, there are some concerns that nettle may interact with conventional medications used for diabetes or high blood pressure, but there are no published reports of such problems occurring.

Safety in those with severe liver or kidney disease has not been established.

Beta-Sitosterol (from *Hypoxis rooperi*)

The South African plant *Hypoxis rooperi* has a long history of native use for bladder and prostate problems. Its tubers contain a family of cholesterol-like compounds called beta-sitosterols, of which the most important is believed to be beta-sitosterolin. In Germany, beta-sitosterol is more widely prescribed for prostate enlargement than saw palmetto.

The scientific evidence for sitosterols is not as strong as that for other BPH treatments widely used in Europe, but there has been at least one solid double-blind study. It followed 200 men with BPH for a period of 6 months.[19] Those treated with sitosterol showed significant improvement in many symptoms of prostate enlargement. Other studies corroborate these results.[20]

The proper dosage of sitosterols should supply 60 mg daily of beta-sitosterol. Full effects may take 6 months to develop.

Detailed safety studies of sitosterol have not been performed, and safety in those with severe kidney or liver disease has not been established. However, no significant side effects have been observed.[21]

Grass Pollen

A special extract of grass pollen is widely used in Europe for the treatment of BPH. While a couple of double-blind studies have found it to be effective, [22,23] the total evidence is weaker than for the treatments just described. Grass pollen extract is just beginning to become available in the United States. Look for products that contain the rye pollen (*Secale cereale*).

Other Natural Treatments for Benign Prostatic Hyperplasia

There are a few other treatments often recommended for BPH, but they lack any real scientific evidence. Pumpkin seeds are approved for use in BPH by Germany's Commission E. The mineral zinc is also commonly recommended in both Europe and the United States as a treatment for prostate disease, as is flax oil. But in the absence of real studies for these treatments I'd suggest sticking with one of the proven herbs above.

BLADDER INFECTION
(Urinary Tract Infection)

Principal Natural Treatments

Cranberry, uva ursi

Other Natural Treatments

Goldenseal, probiotics, vitamin C, zinc, low-sugar diet

Bladder infections are a common problem for women, accounting for more than 6 million office visits each year. Men, because of the greater distance between their bladder and urethral opening, only rarely develop bladder infections.

The primary symptoms of a bladder infection are burning during urination, frequency of urination, and urgency to urinate, possibly accompanied by pain in the lower abdomen and cloudy or bloody urine. Occasionally, the infection spreads upward into the kidneys, producing symptoms such as intense back pain, high fever, chills, nausea, and diarrhea.

Conventional treatment for bladder infections consists of appropriate antibiotic treatment guided by urine culture. At press time, a report was released suggesting that it is appropriate for women with frequent bladder infections to have on hand a prescription for antibiotics for the purpose of self-treatment when symptoms arise. Women who have had extremely frequent bladder infections sometimes take antibiotics continuously to prevent the condition.

Principal Natural Treatments for Bladder Infection

Women who do not want to use antibiotics may be able to find some help through the use of herbs. However, if symptoms do not improve or signs of a kidney infection develop, medical attention is essential to prevent serious complications.

Cranberry: May Help Prevent Infections

Cranberry juice is commonly used to prevent bladder infections as well as to overcome low-level chronic infections. The cranberry plant is a close relative of the common blueberry. Native Americans used it both as food and as a treatment for bladder and kidney diseases. The Pilgrims learned about cranberry from local tribes and quickly adopted it for their own use. Subsequent physicians used it for bladder infections, for "bladder gravel," and to remove "blood toxins."

In the 1920s, researchers observed that drinking cranberry juice makes the urine more acidic. Because common urine infection bacteria such as *E. coli* dislike acid surroundings, physicians concluded that they had discovered a scientific explanation for the traditional uses of cranberry. This discovery led to widespread medical use of cranberry juice for bladder infections. Cranberry fell out of favor after World War II, only to return in the 1960s as a self-treatment for bladder infections.

More recent research has revised the conclusions reached by scientists in the 1920s. It appears that acidification of the urine is not so important as cranberry's ability to interfere with the bacteria establishing a foothold on the bladder wall.[1–4] If the bacteria can't hold on, they will be washed out with the stream of urine. Furthermore, studies suggest that in women who frequently develop bladder infections, bacteria have an especially easy time holding on to the bladder wall.[5]

When taken regularly, cranberry juice may fix this problem and break the cycle of repeated infection. Cranberry juice also seems to be helpful for chronic bladder infections, those that continue for months with few to no symptoms.

What Is the Scientific Evidence for Cranberry?

A 6-month study followed 153 women with an average age of 78.5 years.[6] This study looked at chronic bladder infections rather than acute bladder infections. Chronic bladder infections are relatively common in older women, and may cause few or no symptoms. The evidence suggests that cranberry can eliminate continuing infections.

Half of the participants were given a standard supermarket cranberry cocktail, and the other half were given a placebo drink prepared to look and taste the same. Both treatments contained the same amount of vitamin C, which was important because vitamin C itself may have some antibacterial effects.

Commercial cranberry cocktail is mostly sugar and contains little cranberry juice. It is natural to wonder whether straight cranberry juice would have been more effective. Nonetheless, the results suggest that even cranberry juice cocktail can prevent chronic bladder infections, as well as eliminate ones that have already begun.

There was a 58% lower rate of bacteria in the urine of the women treated with cranberry as compared to those given placebo. Also, if a woman had bacteria in the urine at one point in the study, the chance that she would still have it a month later was 73% lower in the cranberry group.

This study has been criticized for several flaws in its design, especially the method used to analyze the urine. It also doesn't tell us whether regular use of cranberry will prevent ordinary acute bladder infections. Nonetheless, it definitely suggests that cranberry juice does have real potential in the treatment of bladder infections.

Dosage

The proper dosage of dry cranberry juice extract is 300 to 400 mg twice daily. For those people who prefer juice, 8 to 16 ounces daily should be enough. For best effect, use true cranberry juice, not sugary cranberry juice cocktail.

Safety Issues

There are no known risks associated with this food for adults, children, and pregnant or nursing women. However, excessive use of cranberry juice may weaken the effect of slightly alkaline drugs, such as many antidepressants and prescription painkillers, by causing them to be excreted more rapidly in the urine.

Uva Ursi: Appears to Be Effective for Acute Bladder Infections

While cranberry is most often used to prevent bladder infections or to treat simmering chronic infections, uva ursi, also known as *bearberry*, can be used to treat the classic painful, acute bladder infection. Uva ursi has a long history of use for urinary conditions in both America and Europe. Until the development of sulfa antibiotics, its principal active component, arbutin, was frequently prescribed by physicians as a treatment for bladder and kidney infections.

The uva ursi plant is a low-lying evergreen bush whose berries are a favorite of bears, thus the name bearberry. However, it is the leaves that are used medicinally. We do not know for sure how uva ursi works. It appears that the arbutin contained in uva ursi leaves is broken down in the intestine to another chemical, hydroquinone. This is altered a bit by the liver and then sent to the kidneys for excretion.[7] Hydroquinone then acts as an antiseptic in the bladder.

The European Scientific Cooperative on Phytotherapy (ESCOP) is a scientific organization assigned the task of harmonizing herb policy among European countries. ESCOP recommends uva ursi for "uncomplicated infections of the urinary tract such as cystitis when antibiotic treatment is not considered essential."[8]

Warning: This herb is definitely not appropriate for kidney infections. If you develop symptoms such as high fever, chills, nausea, vomiting, diarrhea, or severe back pain, get medical assistance immediately.

Furthermore, hydroquinone can be toxic (see Safety Issues). For this reason it is not a good idea to take uva ursi for a long period of time.

What Is the Scientific Evidence for Uva Ursi?

Surprisingly little research has been done on uva ursi.[9]

Treatment No double-blind studies have evaluated the clinical effectiveness of uva ursi. Two studies evaluated the antibacterial power of the urine of people who were taking uva ursi and found activity against most major bacteria that infect the urinary tract.[10,11]

Prevention One double-blind study followed 57 women for 1 year.[12] Half were given a standardized dose of uva ursi, and the other received placebo. Over the course of the study, none of the women on uva ursi developed a bladder infection, whereas five of the untreated women did. However, most experts do not believe that continuous treatment with uva ursi is a good idea.

Dosage

The dosage of uva ursi should be adjusted to provide 400 to 800 mg of arbutin daily.[13,14,15] This dosage should not be exceeded. If the herb is not successful within 1 week, you should definitely seek medical attention. No more than 2 weeks of treatment with uva ursi is recommended even under medical supervision, and it should not be used more than five times a year. Uva ursi should be taken with meals to minimize gastrointestinal upset.

Interestingly, research suggests that arbutin's antibiotic activity depends on the presence of alkaline urine. Many women take vitamin C during bladder infections to acidify the urine and, it is hoped, inhibit the bacteria. However, this may tend to block the effect of uva ursi. For this reason, it may be counterproductive to use both uva ursi and vitamin C. Conversely, supplements thought to alkalinize the urine may improve uva ursi's effectiveness. These include calcium citrate, calcium gluconate, and baking soda.

Safety Issues

Unfortunately, hydroquinone is a liver toxin, a carcinogen, and an irritant.[16–19] For this reason, uva ursi is not recommended for young children, pregnant or nursing women, and those with severe liver or kidney disease.

However, significant problems are rare among people using uva ursi products in appropriate dosages for a short period of time. Gastrointestinal distress (ranging from mild nausea and diarrhea to vomiting) can occur, especially with prolonged use.[20]

Other Natural Treatments for Bladder Infection

The following treatments are often proposed as treatments for bladder infections, but there is as yet little to no scientific confirmation of their effectiveness.

Goldenseal

The herb goldenseal is widely recommended for bladder infections, based on the antibiotic properties of its ingredient berberine. However, it is not at all clear that after taking goldenseal by mouth enough berberine accumulates in the bladder to do anything.

In the past, herbalists would instill goldenseal preparations directly into the bladder, a process that I do not recommend trying yourself. The safety of goldenseal in young children, pregnant or nursing women, and those with severe liver or kidney disease has not been established.

Probiotics

Probiotics, or "friendly bacteria," particularly those found in live yogurt such as *Lactobacillus acidophilus, Bifidobacterium bifidum* (bifidus for short), and *Lactobacillus bulgaricus,* may also be useful in preventing bladder infections. Many bladder infections are caused by the migration of vaginal and rectal bacteria into the urinary tract. When friendly bacteria are present, pathogenic, or disease-causing, bacteria have a difficult time proliferating. Friendly bacteria may be taken orally or introduced in the form of a douche.

Unfortunately, the quality control of acidophilus supplements seems to be very poor. Unless you have a home microbiology lab, it will be difficult for you to tell whether the acidophilus you are buying is really alive. Live culture yogurt may be preferable, unless your store can supply documentation proving that its acidophilus is still alive at time of purchase.

Other Supplements

Many nutritionally oriented physicians believe that regularly taking vitamin C and zinc supplements, and decreasing sugar in the diet, will help improve immunity against bladder infections.

CANCER PREVENTION
Reducing the Risk

Principal Natural Treatments
Vitamin E, selenium, garlic, tomatoes (lycopene), vitamin C,
green tea, soy

Other Natural Treatments
Folic acid, vitamin D, flaxseed oil (lignans), grapes (resveratrol),
sulforaphane, turmeric, rosemary, licorice, ginseng, bromelain,
melatonin, goldenseal, elagic acid, quercetin, citrus juices, betulin,
papaw tree bark, blue-green algae, probiotics, calcium

Not Recommended Treatments
Beta-carotene

Cancer is the second major cause of death (next to heart disease) in the United States. It claims the lives of more than half a million Americans a year out of the nearly 1.4 million who get the disease. The probability of getting cancer increases with age. Two-thirds of all cases are in people older than 65.[1]

According to the American Cancer Society, one in two men and one in three women will face cancer during their lifetimes. However, it appears that you significantly cut your cancer risk by how you choose to lead your life. That is the bright consensus of an international panel recently convened by the American Institute for Cancer Research and the World Cancer Research Fund.[2]

The panel found four key ways to reduce the odds of getting cancer: Eat the right foods, exercise, watch your weight, and do not smoke. The experts reviewed diet and cancer findings from over 4,500 studies to reach this consensus.

What Causes Cancer?

Cancer is believed to begin with a mutation in a single cell. However, a cell doesn't become cancerous overnight. Several mutations in a row are necessary to create all the characteristic features of cancer. Ordinarily, cells have a self-destruct mechanism that causes them to die when their DNA is damaged. However, in developing cancer cells, something interferes with the self-destruct sequence. It may be that the cancer-causing mutations themselves turn off the countdown.

The DNA alterations that create a cancer cell give it a certain independence from the ordinary rules of cell behavior. Normal cells are highly influenced by nearby cells, with the result that they "get along" well with their neighbors. For example, the growth of a healthy cell is ruled by special growth factors given off by surrounding tissues. However, cancer cells either grow without such growth factors or simply make their own. Many types of cancer cells can also trigger the growth of new blood vessels to feed them.

Cancerous mutations appear to be caused mainly by exposure to carcinogenic substances, of which tobacco is the most common. Many carcinogens exist in the diet as well, such as salt-cured and smoked meats.

Free radicals also appear to play a major role in promoting cancer. These chemically unstable substances are produced by many factors, and are believed to affect heart disease and aging (for more information about free radicals in general, see Atherosclerosis). The best documented natural treatments for preventing cancer have antioxidant properties.

Hormones can also help cancer get a start. For example, a newly formed cancer of the prostate or the breast is stimulated by the hormones that ordinarily control tissue in that part of the body. This is why estrogen-replacement therapy can increase the risk of breast cancer and why estrogen suppression is often recommended for women with a history of breast cancer. Substances found in soy may help reduce the incidence of certain cancers by blocking the effects of estrogen and other hormones.

The key to preventing cancer is to minimize your exposure to carcinogens. Quitting smoking is essential, and reducing your intake of smoked, charred, pickled, and salt-cured meats is also believed to be helpful. Eating a diet that is high in fruits, vegetables, and whole grains and low in saturated fat (found primarily in dairy and meat) also lowers your chance of developing cancer.[3] Vegetables in the broccoli family may be particularly helpful.

When it comes to natural cancer prevention, conventional and natural medicine are converging. The dietary suggestions listed previously were originally championed by "alternative" physicians, but they are all presently mainstream. Furthermore, many of the supplements described here are rapidly entering the mainstream as well.

Because the following material is so complex, I have summarized it in the section titled Putting It All Together. You can skip to it now if you want just the conclusions. You can also read *The Natural Pharmacist Guide to Reducing Cancer Risk.*

Principal Natural Treatments
for Reducing Cancer Risk

It is rather difficult to prove that taking a certain supplement will reduce the chance of developing cancer. You really need enormous long-term studies in which some people are given the supplement while others are given placebo. We do have evidence of this type for vitamin E and selenium. These two supplements definitely appear to lower the risk of certain kinds of cancer.

For other supplements, the evidence is more circumstantial. Observational studies have found that people who happen to take in high levels of certain vitamins or herbs in their diets develop a lower incidence of specific cancers. These results are less reliable because such people may also have other healthy lifestyle habits. Researchers attempt to factor out these other influences, however.

Evidence of this type suggests that the herb garlic may reduce the odds of cancer, perhaps because it contains a lot of selenium. Vitamin C supplements do not appear to be very effective, but a substantial intake of vitamin C and beta-carotene in the form of fruits and vegetables does seem to reduce the incidence of cancer significantly. Beta-carotene taken as a supplement may actually be harmful.

Vitamin E: Probably Reduces the Odds of Several Types of Cancer

Vitamin E has the best evidence behind it of any supplement suggested as a preventive treatment for cancer.

In an intervention trial (see Atherosclerosis for the definition of an intervention trial) that involved 29,133 smokers, those who were given 50 mg of vitamin E daily for 5 to 8 years showed a 32% reduction in the incidence of prostate cancer and a 41% drop in prostate cancer deaths.[4] Surprisingly, results were seen soon after the beginning of supplementation. This was unexpected because prostate cancer grows very slowly. A cancer that shows up today actually started to develop many years ago. The fact that vitamin E almost immediately lowered the incidence of prostate cancer suggests that it somehow blocks the step at which a hidden prostate cancer makes the leap to being detectable.

The same study also showed that vitamin E supplementation reduced colon cancer by 16%.

The dose of vitamin E used in this study, which corresponds to about 50 to 75 IU of vitamin E, is lower than is usually recommended. It is quite reasonable to assume that a higher dose would be more effective, although this has not been proven.

Observational studies have also shown benefit. Researchers at the Fred Hutchinson Cancer Research Center in Seattle determined that supplemental vitamin E (200 IU or more daily) cut colon cancer risk by 57%.[5,6] Other studies have shown reductions ranging from 29 to 68%, depending on the length of time the participants used vitamin E, as well as other factors.[7,8]

Similarly good results have been seen in stomach cancer; mouth, throat, and laryngeal cancer; and liver cancer.[9–12] However, vitamin E does not appear to be strongly effective against lung cancer.[13]

Vitamin E is typically supplemented at a dose of 400 to 800 IU daily. Realistically, you can't get this much vitamin E in your diet, so supplements are necessary.

Vitamin E is generally believed to be safe at this dosage level. However vitamin E is known to affect blood clotting, and for this reason should not be combined with aspirin or prescription blood thinners except under a physician's supervision.[14] Vitamin E may also present some risk of bleeding on its own. In one study, vitamin E supplementation was associated with an increase in hemorrhagic stroke, the kind of stroke caused by bleeding.[15] For this reason, doses above 800 IU daily should only be used on the advice of a physician.

Selenium: May Protect Against Lung, Prostate, and Colon Cancer

It has long been known that severe selenium deficiency increases the risk of cancer.[16] However, by itself, this does not prove that taking selenium supplements will make a difference if you are not deficient in it.

A recent double-blind study did find that selenium supplements can dramatically reduce the incidence of cancer. The results were so impressive they caught the researchers by surprise. The study was actually designed to detect selenium's effects on skin cancer.[17] It followed 1,312 individuals, half of whom were given 200 mcg of selenium daily. The participants were treated for an average of 2.8 years and were followed for about 6 years. Although no significant effect on skin cancer was found, the researchers were startled when the results showed that people taking selenium had a 50% reduction in cancer deaths and a 37% decrease in cancer of the lung, colon, and prostate. The findings were so remarkable that the researchers felt obliged to break the blind and allow all the participants to take selenium. However, further research needs to be done to confirm these findings. In a disease such as cancer, very large and long-term studies are necessary to be sure of the results.

The recommended dosage of selenium is 50 to 200 mcg daily. In children, this may be reduced to 1.5 mcg per pound body weight. Of the various sources of selenium, organic forms, such as selenomethionine, selenium-rich yeast, and selenium-enriched garlic, may be preferable to inorganic sodium selenite.

When taken at the recommended dosage, selenium is believed to be safe and side-effect free. Long-term use of selenium at a level of 200 mcg daily has been shown to be safe in adults, and doses up to 350 mcg daily are believed to be harmless.[18] Toxic effects begin to be seen at levels of 750 to 1,000 mcg daily, and include gastrointestinal distress, central nervous system changes, garlic-like breath odor, and loss of hair and fingernails.

Maximum safe dosages in young children, pregnant or nursing women, and those with severe liver or kidney disease has not been established.

Garlic: May Reduce the Risk of Colon Cancer

A great deal of evidence from observational studies (see Atherosclerosis for the definition of an observational study) suggests that garlic may help prevent cancer.

In the Iowa Women's Study, a very large and well-conducted observational study, women who ate significant amounts of garlic were found to be about 30% less likely to develop colon cancer.[19] Similar results were seen in other observational studies performed in China, Italy, and the United States.[20,21]

We do not know for sure how garlic might work to prevent cancer. Like vitamin E, whole garlic possesses antioxidant properties.[22,23] Furthermore, various garlic extracts have also been shown to suppress the known DNA-damaging activity of several drugs and toxins.[24] Finally, garlic contains high levels of selenium, which is thought to reduce the risk of cancer (see the previous discussion under Selenium).[25]

It's unclear how much garlic is needed for a cancer-preventive effect, but one or two cloves daily should probably suffice. Side effects (other than bad breath) are rare, and garlic is on the FDA's list of agents that are generally regarded as safe. However, raw garlic in excessive doses can cause stomach upset, heartburn, nausea and vomiting, diarrhea, facial flushing, rapid heartbeat, and insomnia. Garlic appears to interfere with blood clotting, so it should not be combined with blood-thinning drugs such as Coumadin (warfarin), Trental (pentoxifylline), or even aspirin except under medical supervision, nor should it be taken around the time of surgery or labor and delivery. There might also be some risk involved in combining garlic with other blood-thinning herbs or natural supplements, such as gingko and high-dose vitamin E, although no problems have been reported.

Beta-Carotene: Helpful in the
Diet, Harmful As a Supplement?

In the early 1980s, a review of the observational studies clearly showed that people whose diets are high in fruits and vegetables have a significantly decreased risk for cancer.[26,27] Some of the strongest evidence relates to lung cancer, for which a high intake of fruits and vegetables was associated with as much as a 70% reduced risk.

Scientists then set about trying to identify the active principle in fruits and vegetables. One group of substances widely available in these foods are carotenes (named after carrots). A careful examination of the data suggests that the level of carotenes in the diet is strongly connected with protection against lung cancer.[28] Evidence also suggests that carotenes protect against bladder cancer,[29] breast cancer,[30] esophageal cancer,[31] and stomach cancer.[32]

The best-known carotene is beta-carotene, a strong antioxidant that the body can convert to vitamin A. It was a natural step to assume that it was the beta-carotene in these foods that was making the difference. In animal studies, beta-carotene supplements seemed to significantly reduce the incidence of cancer.[33] Unfortunately, studies in which people were actually given beta-carotene supplements (rather than foods containing it) have not shown wonderful results.

The anticancer bubble burst for beta-carotene in 1994 when the results of the Alpha-Tocopherol, Beta-Carotene (ATBC) study came in. Apparently, beta-carotene did not prevent but actually *increased* the risk of getting lung cancer by 18%. This intervention trial had followed 29,133 male smokers in Finland who took supplements of either 50 mg of vitamin E (alpha-tocopherol) or 20 mg of beta-carotene, or both, or a placebo daily for 5 to 8 years.[34] This was the same study mentioned previously in which vitamin E reduced the risk of prostate and colon cancer; however, beta-carotene worked in the opposite direction.

In January 1996, researchers monitoring the Beta-Carotene and Retinol Efficacy Trial (CARET) confirmed this bad news with more of their own: The beta-carotene group had 46% more cases of lung cancer deaths.[35] This study involved smokers, former smokers, and workers exposed to asbestos.

Alarmed, the National Cancer Institute (NCI) pushed the brake pedal on the $42 million trial 21 months before it was finished. At about the same time, the 12-year Physicians' Health Study of 22,000 male physicians was finding that 50 mg of beta-carotene taken every other day had no effect at all—good or bad—on the risk of cancer or heart disease.[36] In this study, 11% of the participants were smokers, and 39% were ex-smokers.

Interestingly, in both the ATBC study and the CARET study, higher levels of carotene intake from the diet *were* associated with lower levels of cancer. Apparently, beta-carotene is not effective alone. Other carotenes found in fruits and vegetables appear to be more important for preventing cancer (see, for example, Lycopene following). It is possible that taking beta-carotene depletes the body of other carotenes, thereby producing an overall harmful effect.[37]

These studies also found that beta-carotene supplements may increase the risk of heart disease and stroke as well. Therefore, I recommend getting your beta-carotene from foods, rather than supplements. The best dietary sources of carotenes are yellow-orange vegetables and dark-green vegetables.

Tomatoes (Lycopene): May Be
More Important Than Beta-Carotene

Lycopene, a carotenoid like beta-carotene, is found in high levels in tomatoes and pink grapefruit. Lycopene appears to exhibit about twice the antioxidant activity of beta-carotene and may be more important for preventing cancer than the better known vitamin.

In one study, elderly Americans consuming a diet high in tomatoes reduced their risk for cancers by 50%.[38] Men and women who ate at least seven servings of tomatoes weekly developed less stomach and colorectal cancers compared to those who ate only two servings weekly.

In another study, 47,894 men were followed for 4 years in an observational study looking for influences on prostate cancer.[39] Their diets were evaluated on the basis of how often they ate fruits, vegetables, and foods containing fruits and vegetables. High levels of tomatoes, tomato sauce, and pizza in the diet were strongly connected to the prevention of prostate cancer. After an evaluation of known nutritional factors in these foods as compared to other foods, lycopene appeared to be the common denominator. Additional impetus has been given to this idea by the discovery of lycopene in reasonably high levels in the human prostate.[40]

Cooked tomatoes appear to be more bioavailable (more readily used by the body) than raw tomatoes, especially when the tomatoes are cooked in oil. Tomato juice does not seem to be helpful.

Vitamin C: Helpful in the Diet,
Not Helpful As a Supplement?

As with beta-carotene, most of the positive studies of vitamin C and cancer prevention have looked at the effect of vitamin C in the diet rather than at actual vitamin C supplements. It is possible the other plant substances that come along with vitamin C are equally or more important. Studies involving vitamin C supplements have not produced stellar results.

Several studies have found a strong association between high dietary vitamin C intake and a reduced incidence of stomach cancer.[41,42,43] One way in which vitamin C may work is by preventing the formation of carcinogenic substances known as N-nitroso compounds in the stomach.

Evidence also suggests that vitamin C from food may also provide a protective effect in colon, esophageal, laryngeal, bladder, cervical, rectal, breast, and perhaps lung cancer.[44–48] However, dietary vitamin C intake does not appear to be associated with protection against prostate cancer.[49]

A few studies have used supplemental vitamin C instead of dietary vitamin C. One found that vitamin C supplementation at 500 mg or more daily was associated with a lower incidence of bladder cancer.[50] However, another study found no connection.[51]

Supplemental vitamin C at 1 g daily failed to prevent new colon cancers after one colon cancer had developed.[52] In another large observational study, 500 mg or more of vitamin C daily over a period of 6 years provided no significant protection against breast cancer.[53] Another study found similar results.[54]

Thus, just as with beta-carotene, it may be that the natural dietary substances that come along with vitamin C are more important for cancer prevention than the vitamin alone. In this case, water-soluble flavonoids may be responsible for the benefit. Eat your fruits and vegetables!

Green Tea: May Help Prevent Many Types of Cancer

Both green tea and black tea come from the tea plant called *Camellia sinensis,* which has been cultivated in China for centuries. The key difference between the two is in preparation. For black tea, the leaves are allowed to oxidize, a process believed to lessen the potency of therapeutic compounds known as polyphenols. Green tea is made by lightly steaming the freshly cut leaf, a process that prevents oxidation and possibly preserves more of the therapeutic effects.

Laboratory and animal studies suggest that tea consumption protects against cancers of the stomach, lung, esophagus, duodenum, pancreas, liver, breast, and colon.[55] A 1994 study of skin cancer in mice found that both black and green teas, even decaffeinated versions, inhibited skin cancer in mice exposed to ultraviolet light and other carcinogens.[56,57] After 31 weeks, mice given the teas brewed at the same concentration humans drink had 72 to 93% fewer skin tumors than mice given only water.

However, results from human studies have not been so clear-cut—some have shown a protective effect, and others have not. Nonetheless, the overall weight of the evidence does lean toward the positive side.[58]

One study followed 8,552 Japanese adults for 9 years.[59] Women who drank more than 10 cups daily had a delay in the onset of cancer and also a 43% lower total rate of cancer occurrence. Males had a 32% lower cancer incidence, but this finding was not statistically significant.

A study in Shanghai, China, found that those who drank green tea had significant reductions in the risk of developing cancers of the rectum and pancreas. No significant decrease in colon cancer was found.[60] A total of 3,818 residents aged 30 to 74 were included in the population study. For men, those who drank the most tea had a 28% lower incidence of rectal cancer and a 37% lower incidence of pancreatic cancer compared to those who did not drink tea regularly. For women, the respective reductions in cancer frequency were even greater: 43% and 47%.

Another study in Shanghai found similar results for stomach cancer. Green tea drinkers were 29% less likely to get stomach cancer than nondrinkers, with those drinking the most tea having the least risk.[61] Interestingly, the risk of stomach cancer did not depend on the person's age at which he or she started drinking green tea. Researchers suggested at which green tea may disrupt the cancer process at both the intermediate and the late stage.

However, this is a rapidly evolving field, and at press time new information has been released suggesting that there were significant flaws in the green tea studies just described. Other recent evidence indicates that black tea may be more protective than green tea. I suggest talking to your physician about the latest information.

The active ingredients in green tea are believed to be polyphenols, especially one known as epigallocatechin gallate (EGCG). Like vitamin C, polyphenols may block the formation of nitrosamines and other cancer-causing compounds and may trap or detoxify carcinogens.[62] Green tea may also exert an estrogen-blocking effect that is helpful in breast and uterine cancer.[63]

The optimum dosage of green tea is unknown. However, you might want to use the amount correlated with good results in the observational studies. That would mean either drinking 3 cups of green tea daily or taking 300 to 400 mg daily of a green tea extract standardized for 80% total polyphenols and 55% epigallocatechin content.

No significant side effects are associated with green tea, other than those due to its (rather low) caffeine content.

Soy: May Reduce the Risk of Hormone-Related Cancers

In many animal studies, soy or soy extracts decreased cancer risk, and observational studies show that the same effect may occur in people as well.[64–67] According to the data that we have, soy may be active against hormone-related cancers such as prostate, breast, and uterine cancer.

Soybeans provide estrogen-like compounds known as *isoflavones*, especially genistein and daidzein. These substances bind to the same sites in the body as estrogen, occupying these sites and keeping natural estrogen away. Estrogen stimulates certain forms of cancer, but soy estrogens exert a milder estrogen-like effect that may not stimulate cancer as much as natural estrogen. This may partially explain soy's apparent protective effect.[68,69] Soy or soy extracts may also affect cancers in other ways, but more remains to be discovered.

However, in observational studies, it is difficult to tell whether the soy is exerting a directly positive effect on its own or whether some of the benefit is due to the fact that people who eat more soy also eat less meat. For more definitive results, we need studies in which soy or soy extracts are added to the diets of a large group of people while another group is given placebo treatment. Unfortunately, this type of research has not yet been performed.

One or two tofu "burgers" or cups of soy milk daily may be enough to produce a beneficial effect. Soy foods are believed to be safe, although high doses of soy can interfere with mineral absorption. There is also some concern that soy may not be advisable for women who have already had breast cancer.

You can also take isolated soy isoflavones. A dosage of 40 to 60 mg daily comes pretty close to dietary intake.

Other Natural Treatments for Reducing Cancer Risk

The substances mentioned in this section have less evidence behind them than the antioxidants just discussed. However, this is a rapidly growing field. By the time you read this book, new information will undoubtedly be available.

Folic Acid

Folic acid deficiency may predispose individuals toward developing cervical cancer,[70] colon cancer,[71,72] lung cancer,[73] and mouth cancer.[74] However, we know very little about whether taking folic acid supplements will help prevent these diseases.

Nonetheless, a deficiency of this essential vitamin is quite common, and if you don't eat a lot of dark-green, leafy vegetables, you will probably find overall benefits from a bit of folic acid supplementation.

A typical dosage is 400 to 800 mcg daily. Folic acid is safe, but because it can mask vitamin B_{12} deficiency, it is wise to get your B_{12} level checked before taking high doses (800 mcg or more).

Vitamin D

Dietary vitamin D intake was connected to a lower rate of occurrence of colon cancer in some studies,[75] but not in others.[76] Do not take more than about 600 IU of vitamin D daily except on the advice of a physician.

Several studies have shown that women who receive less sunlight develop more breast cancer. Because sunlight produces vitamin D, it has been suggested that vitamin D may prevent breast cancer, but this is just speculation.

Flaxseed Oil (Lignans)

Substances known as *lignans* are found in several foods and may produce anticancer benefits. They are converted in the digestive tract to estrogen-like substances known as enterolactone and enterodiol.[77] Like soy isoflavones (see the previous discussion under Soy), these substances prevent estrogen from attaching to cells and may thereby block its cancer-promoting effects.

Lignans are found most abundantly in flaxseed, a high-fiber grain that has been cultivated since ancient Egyptian times. Flaxseed oil is also a rich source of an omega-3 fatty acid: alpha-linolenic acid.

Studies in humans and animals suggest that lignans may provide anticancer protection, especially against breast cancer.[78] However, this evidence is not strong.

Weak evidence also suggests that the alpha-linolenic acid in flaxseed oil may act against breast cancer. Low levels of alpha-linolenic acid in breast fatty tissues were associated with an increase in cancer and its spread (metastasis) to other areas of the body.[79]

The optimum dose of flaxseed oil is not known. The typical supplemental dosage recommended by some nutritionists is 1 to 2 tablespoons daily. Flaxseed oil is easily damaged by heat and light, so do not cook with it. The most palatable way to take it is by adding it to foods, such as using it as a salad dressing. Flaxseed oil is believed to be safe, although it occasionally causes constipation.

Grapes (Resveratrol)

Resveratrol is a phytochemical found in at least 72 different plants, including mulberries and peanuts. Grapes are its richest source. Red wine, which is made from grapes, contains a lot of resveratrol, which may account for some of the beneficial effects attributed to wine in some studies.

Resveratrol is an antioxidant with intriguing anticancer effects as determined in test-tube studies.[80] However, little direct evidence supports the idea that resveratrol is helpful. The proper dosage is not known, and safety studies have not yet been completed. In addition, researchers have been unable to measure significant levels of resveratrol in the bloodstream of subjects that had drank several glasses of red wine, suggesting the resveratrol is not bioavailable, or easily absorbed by the body, to any extent.[81]

Other Treatments on the Horizon

Provocative evidence suggests that a substance called sulforaphane, found in broccoli and related vegetables, may possess anticancer properties. Recently, broccoli sprouts have been touted as a cancer treatment on the basis of their high content of sulforaphane. However, this recommendation is still highly speculative.

Weak or indirect evidence also suggests some cancer-preventive benefits for the spices turmeric and rosemary as well as for licorice, ginseng, bromelain, melatonin, goldenseal, elagic acid (from grapes, raspberries, strawberries, apples, walnuts, and pecans), quercetin (a bioflavonoid found in many foods, including apples), citrus juices, betulin (from white birch tree), papaw tree bark, blue-green algae, and probiotics ("friendly" bacteria, such as acidophilus).

It has been suggested that calcium supplementation can reduce the risk of colon cancer, but after researchers took a closer look at the data, this supposition did not hold up.[82]

Putting It All Together

To prevent cancer, the best thing you can do for yourself is eat a diet high in fruits and vegetables and whole grains and low in smoked, charred, pickled, and salt-cured meats as well as other animal products. Increasing exercise and losing weight also appears to help significantly, and stopping smoking is essential.

The strongest evidence for any supplement in the treatment of cancer concerns vitamin E and prostate cancer. Vitamin E also seems to reduce the incidence of other cancers, especially stomach cancer; mouth, throat, and laryngeal cancer; and liver cancer. A typical dosage is 400 IU daily of alpha-tocopherol.

Selenium supplementation (200 mcg daily) appears to be helpful for preventing lung, colon, and prostate cancers.

Garlic appears to help prevent colon cancer.

Purified beta-carotene has not been shown to prevent cancer (and it may even increase the risk), but carotenes in the diet appear to protect against lung cancer as well as bladder cancer, breast cancer, stomach cancer, and cancer of the upper digestive tract.

Tomatoes seem to reduce the occurrence of prostate cancer as well as stomach and colon cancer, perhaps due to their content of the natural carotene lycopene. Cooked tomatoes appear to be more bioavailable (more readily used by the body) than raw tomatoes, especially when the tomatoes are cooked in oil.

Green tea may help prevent colon cancer, and weaker evidence suggests that it may help prevent cancer of the stomach, small intestine, pancreas, lungs, breast, and uterus.

Soy may help prevent hormone-sensitive cancers, such as those of the breast, prostate, uterus, and colon.

Little direct evidence supports the idea that vitamin C supplements prevent cancer, but foods high in vitamin C seem to lower the incidence of stomach cancer as well as colon, esophageal, laryngeal, bladder, cervical, rectal, and breast cancer.

Folic acid deficiency appears to be associated with cervical, colon, lung, and mouth cancer, but whether taking extra folic acid will help has not been determined.

Please refer to the chapter to learn about safety issues associated with some of these substances.

"CANDIDA"

Principal Natural Treatments

There are no well-established natural treatments for "candida."

Other Natural Treatments

Probiotics, capryllic acid, grapefruit seed extract, betaine hydrochloride, peppermint oil, oregano oil, lavender oil, tea tree oil, barberry, red thyme, pau d'arco, garlic, low-sugar diet, avoid foods with high mold content

---

Candida albicans is a naturally occurring yeast that flourishes in moist areas, such as the digestive tract, the vagina, and skin folds. Ordinarily, its population is kept in check by bacteria that live in the same areas. When normal bacteria are disturbed by antibiotics, however, yeast populations can grow to abnormally high levels.

For women, the most common symptom of excess candida is a vaginal yeast infection, as marked by itchiness, redness, burning on urination, and a yeasty odor. However, candida can also overpopulate in the mouth (thrush), in the warm moist environment under a diaper (diaper rash), and in other areas.

Candida usually confines itself to the surface of mucous membranes and does not penetrate deeply into the body. However, in people whose immune systems are severely depressed, such as those with AIDS or leukemia, candida can become a dangerous, invasive organism. The medical name for this rare and dire condition is *systemic candidiasis.*

Besides this official meaning, systemic candidiasis has another meaning that was coined in the world of alternative medicine. As used there, it is a loose term connoting a whole syndrome of symptoms believed to be related to candida. Equivalent terms are *chronic candida,* the *yeast syndrome,* the *yeast hypersensitivity syndrome* (my favorite), or just plain *Candida* for short.

Conventional medicine does not recognize the existence of this alternative syndrome. However, for several years it was practically impossible to walk into an alternative practitioner's office and not walk out with the diagnosis of candida. Fortunately, this excess enthusiasm has cooled in recent years. Among people who believe that they have a candida problem, perhaps 1 in 20 will benefit significantly from treatment for it. Candida is more a fad than a reality. Nonetheless, it has some reality behind it as well.

The story of "the yeast syndrome" begins in 1983, when Orion Truss published *The Missing Diagnosis*. This was followed by William Crook's much more famous *The Yeast Connection*. These books claim that a person who is chronically colonized by too much candida may develop an allergy-like hypersensitivity to it. The symptoms of this allergy are said to be similar to those of other allergies, including sinus congestion, fatigue, intestinal gas, difficulty concentrating, depression, muscle aches, and many other common complaints.

The regimen outlined by Dr. Crook consists of two parts: treatments that tend toward diminishing the total body burden of candida; and less convincing recommendations that attempt to lessen allergic reactions toward yeast in general.

To decrease the amount of yeast in the body, Dr. Crook recommends avoiding certain substances, including antibiotics, corticosteroids, birth control pills, sugar, and most sweet foods (it is his contention that dietary sugar "feeds yeast"). He also recommends the use of various supplements and even strong prescription drugs to directly kill yeast or at least interfere with its growth.

Next, Dr. Crook recommends avoiding foods containing yeast of any type, for he believes that those who are allergic to candida will also be allergic to other members of the fungus family. Thus Dr. Crook forbids fermented foods, such as beer, cheese, breads containing baker's yeast, tomato paste (which has a significant mold content), and even mushrooms.

Some of these recommendations seem far-fetched. Although both mushrooms and candida fall into the broad category of fungi, they are not very closely related. Cats and elephants are both mammals, for example, but an allergy to one does not generally imply an allergy to the other. It is difficult to believe that those with sensitivity to candida should also cross-react with food mushrooms, and I have seldom seen it in real life.

Similarly, candida and baker's yeast bear only a distant relationship. Although many people with apparent candida problems do in fact react negatively to bread, it may not be the yeast in the bread that is causing the problem. People with allergies to candida are basically highly allergenic people. They may simply be allergic to the wheat in bread rather than to the yeast. After all, wheat is the second most common food allergen.

There is no conventional medical treatment for yeast hypersensitivity syndrome because conventional medicine does not recognize its existence.

Natural Treatments for Candida

There is no scientific evidence that any treatment can reduce the symptoms caused by oversensitivity to candida.

Many treatments can reduce the amount of yeast in the body, and people with a genuine allergy to candida may feel better once this is achieved. Unfortunately, it isn't possible to eliminate *Candida albicans* permanently. No matter how successful a treatment may be, as soon as it is stopped, candida will return. It has to because it is a natural inhabitant of the body. However, we know from other conditions, such as vaginal yeast infections, that sufficient intake of probiotics, or "friendly bacteria," can help keep yeast regrowth within reasonable bounds. It is probably best to use a mixture of organisms, including acidophilus, bulgaricus, and bifidus. The daily dose should provide 1 to 10 billion viable organisms.

Agents that may reduce the amount of yeast in the body include capryllic acid, grapefruit seed extract, betaine hydrochloride, peppermint oil, oregano oil, lavender oil, tea tree oil, barberry, red thyme, pau d'arco, and garlic. However, the scientific foundation for the use of these treatments is weak, and the appropriate dosage of each has not been determined. Some of these treatments may be toxic if taken to excess or for prolonged periods.

Other Treatments

As mentioned earlier, proponents of the candida syndrome further believe that it is important to restrict sugar in the diet, even fruit sugar. This concept is based on the idea that "sugar feeds yeast." However, there is no scientific evidence that dietary sugar increases the growth of candida. They also recommend eliminating all foods with high mold content, such as alcoholic drinks, peanuts, cheeses, bread, and dried fruits. Although these foods cannot increase the amount of candida in your body, they contain yeasts that you could conceivably be allergic to.

CANKER SORES

Principal Natural Treatments

Deglycyrrhizinated licorice

Canker sores are small ulcers in the mouth caused by an assortment of viruses. A susceptibility to canker sores tends to run in families. No successful conventional treatment is available.

Principal Natural Treatments for Canker Sores

A chemically altered form of licorice known as deglyc-yrrhizinated licorice (DGL) may be useful in canker sores.

DGL adheres to inflamed mucous membranes, which has made it a useful treatment for ulcers (see the discussion of DGL under Ulcers). Although no good scientific evidence supports the use of DGL for canker sores, many people report impressive and rapid relief of their symptoms after taking it.[1] Pain levels noticeably decrease within minutes, and remain reduced for hours. According to anecdotal reports, frequent use of DGL throughout the day can almost entirely eliminate the discomfort of canker sores.

This form of licorice is believed to be safe, although safety has not been established in young children, pregnant or nursing women, and those with severe liver or kidney disease. The main problem with DGL is that it must be sucked to coat the canker sores, and some people find its taste objectionable.

CARDIOMYOPATHY

Principal Natural Treatments

Coenzyme Q_{10}, carnitine

Cardiomyopathy is a little understood condition in which the muscle tissue of the heart becomes diseased. There are several distinct forms of cardiomyopathy that may or may not be similar in origin. Medical treatment consists mainly of medications that attempt to compensate for the increasing failure of the heart to function properly. A heart transplant may ultimately be necessary.

Principal Natural Treatments for Cardiomyopathy

Cardiomyopathy is certainly not a disease that you should treat yourself! For this reason, I deliberately do not discuss dosage or safety issues in this section. However, in consultation with your physician, you may want to consider adding the following two supplements to your treatment regimen.

Coenzyme Q_{10}

There is good evidence that the naturally occurring substance coenzyme Q_{10} (CoQ_{10}) is beneficial in some forms of cardiomyopathy.[1,2,3] (For more details about CoQ_{10}, see Congestive Heart Failure).

In a 6-year trial, 143 people with moderately severe cardiomyopathy were given CoQ_{10} daily in addition to standard medical care.[4] The results showed a significant improvement in cardiac function (technically, *ejection fraction*) in 84% of the study participants. Most of them improved by several stages on a scale that measures the severity of heart failure (technically, *NYHA class*). Furthermore, a comparison with individuals on conventional therapy alone appeared to show a reduction in mortality.

This study was an open trial, meaning that participants knew that they were being treated. As explained in the introduction, such studies are not fully reliable due to the power of suggestion. However, these results, including objective measurements of heart function, were so impressive that it is hard to believe the power of suggestion alone could explain them. Nonetheless, double-blind studies are more definitive.

There have been a few such studies of CoQ_{10} in cardiomyopathy. One double-blind controlled trial followed 80 people with various forms of cardiomyopathy over a period of 3 years.[5] Of those treated with CoQ_{10}, 89% improved significantly, but when the treatment was stopped, their heart function deteriorated.

No benefit was seen in another double-blind study, but it was a smaller and shorter trial and enrolled only people who had one particular type of cardiomyopathy (idiopathic dilated cardiomyopathy).[6]

Carnitine

There is a little evidence that the vitamin-like supplement carnitine may be useful in cardiomyopathy.[7,8] Carnitine is believed to work well with CoQ_{10}, and the two treatments are often combined.[9] (For more information on carnitine, see *The Natural Pharmacist: Your Complete Guide to Vitamins and Supplements*.)

CATARACTS
(Prevention)

Principal Natural Treatments
Vitamin C, vitamin E, dietary carotenes

Other Natural Treatments
Bilberry, ginkgo, grape seed PCOs, turmeric, zinc, riboflavin, methionine, cysteine, melatonin

---

Cataracts—an opaque buildup of damaged proteins in the lens of the eye—are the leading cause of visual decline in those over 65. In fact, most people in that age group have at least the beginnings of cataract formation. Many factors contribute to the development of cataracts but damage by free radicals is believed to play a major role. (See Athero-sclerosis for a description of free radicals.)

Cataracts can be removed surgically. Although this has become a relatively quick, safe, easy, and painless surgery, it does not result in completely normal vision. Clearly, preventing cataracts, if possible, would be preferable.

Principal Natural Treatments
for Cataract Prevention

Evidence suggests that various antioxidants may help prevent cataracts.

Vitamin C

In an observational study of 50,800 nurses who were followed for 8 years, a history of taking vitamin C supplements for more than 10 years was associated with a 45% lower risk of cataracts.[1]

Interestingly, diets high in vitamin C were not found to be protective—only supplemental vitamin C made a difference. This is the opposite of what has been found with vitamin C in the prevention of other diseases (see the discussions of vitamin C under Atherosclerosis and Cancer).

Vitamin C is generally believed to be quite safe, at least at dosages up to 500 mg daily. It is often stated that that long-term use of vitamin C can cause kidney stones, but in the large-scale Harvard Prospective Health Professional Follow-Up Study, those taking the most vitamin C (over 1,500 mg daily) had a lower risk of kidney stones than those taking the least amounts.[2] Nonetheless, individuals with a history of kidney stones and those with kidney failure should probably restrict daily vitamin C intake to about 100 mg daily. Taking more than 1,000 mg daily of vitamin C can deplete the body's copper stores, so taking 1 to 3 mg of copper daily as a supplement may be advisable.

Vitamin E

According to observational studies (not as large as the one described under vitamin C) researchers have found that foods high in vitamin E, as well as vitamin E supplements, are associated with a reduced risk of cataracts.[3–8] These results are corroborated by a study in animals.[9]

A typical dosage of vitamin E is 400 IU daily. Vitamin E is generally believed to be safe at this dose. However, in one study, vitamin E supplementation was associated with an increase in hemorrhagic stroke, the kind of stroke caused by bleeding.[10] Considering its ability to reduce blood clotting, vitamin E should not be taken by those with bleeding problems, or combined with aspirin or prescription blood thinners, such as Coumadin (warfarin) and Trental (pentoxifylline), except under a physician's supervision.[11] There also might conceivably be potential risks in combining vitamin E with other natural substances known to thin the blood, such as garlic and ginkgo, although no problems have been reported.

Carotenes

Foods high in carotenes appear to protect against cataract formation.[12,13] In these studies, lutein (found in dark-green vegetables) seemed to be especially helpful for women, whereas the type of carotenes found in carrots was more helpful in men. Lycopene, a carotene found in tomatoes, was associated with a reduced occurrence of cataracts in both sexes.

However, taking the supplement beta-carotene by itself does not appear to be protective.[14,15] This is one more strike against this antioxidant, which has failed to prove beneficial in other conditions as well (see the discussions of beta-carotene under Atherosclerosis and Cancer).

Other Natural Treatments for Cataract Prevention

Herbs high in antioxidant flavonoids may also be helpful in protecting against cataracts. The ones most commonly mentioned include bilberry, ginkgo, proanthocyanidins (PCOs) from grape seed, and turmeric. However, of these, only bilberry has any direct evidence in its favor, and that evidence is weak.[16]

Bilberry is a commonly eaten food and as such is believed to be safe, although safety in young children, pregnant or nursing women, and those with severe kidney or liver disease has not been established. People using blood thinners, such as Coumadin (warfarin), Trental (pentoxifylline), or even aspirin, should not use bilberry without consulting a physician.

The supplements zinc, riboflavin, methionine, cysteine, and melatonin are frequently mentioned as helpful for preventing cataracts, but the evidence that they really work is slim to nonexistent.

CERVICAL DYSPLASIA

Principal Natural Treatments
There are no well-established natural treatments for cervical dysplasia.

Other Natural Treatments
Folic acid (for women on oral contraceptives), multivitamin and mineral supplement, "emmenagogue herbs" (squaw vine, motherwort, true unicorn, false unicorn, black cohosh, blessed thistle)

Very few cancers can be identified so far ahead of the danger point as cancer of the cervix. The cells lining the surface of the cervix begin to show changes visible under a microscope a decade or more before invasive cancer develops, in plenty of time for definitive treatment. For this reason, a regular, properly performed and interpreted Pap smear is one of medicine's most effective preventive methods.

The stages of progression from a healthy cervix to cancer begin with what is called mild dysplasia: precancerous alterations in structure and activity. Subsequently, altered cells spread from the surface of the cervix down toward the underlying tissue. In the early stages, cancerous changes may disappear on their own, but once these cells fully penetrate the lining, progression to true cancer usually occurs within 5 to 10 years.

Medical treatment consists of watchful waiting for spontaneous regression during the early stages and more aggressive removal of the cervical lining by laser, freezing, or other techniques if no regression occurs. These options are usually successful; however, they are invasive and frequently uncomfortable.

Natural Treatments for Cervical Dysplasia

It has been claimed that various natural herbs and supplements can improve the odds of early stages of dysplasia changing back to normal cells. If your physician suggests watchful waiting and a repeat examination, it should be safe to try some of these methods during the waiting period. However, there is no real scientific evidence that these treatments are effective, and in all circumstances close medical supervision is necessary to verify good results or identify failure. Alternative treatment is definitely not advisable for severe cervical dysplasia.

Folic Acid

Folic acid deficiency appears to increase the ease with which cervical cancer can develop. Studies have also found that high doses of folic acid, far above nutritional needs, can help reverse cervical dysplasia in women taking oral contraceptives but not in the population at large.[1–4] However, these findings have been disputed.

The dosage of folic acid used for treatment purposes is often as much as 10 mg daily. Because folic acid can mask vitamin B_{12} deficiency, dosages at this level must be prescribed by a physician. Possible side effects include nausea, flatulence, and loss of appetite as well as an increased rate of seizures in epileptics. The safety of high doses of folic acid in young children, pregnant or nursing women, and those with severe kidney or liver disease has not been established.

General Nutritional Support

Studies have found that women with cervical dysplasia tend to show a high frequency of general nutritional deficiencies, as high as 67% in one survey.[5] For this reason, it probably makes sense to take a multivitamin and mineral supplement. Particular vitamins most commonly associated with cervical dysplasia when deficient include beta-carotene, vitamin C, vitamin B_6, selenium, and folic acid.[6,7]

Emmenagogues

Many practitioners of herbal medicine feel that a class of herbs known as emmenagogues can be helpful in cervical dysplasia. These include squaw vine, motherwort, true unicorn, false unicorn, black cohosh, and blessed thistle.

CHOLESTEROL
(Elevated)

Principal Natural Treatments
Garlic, red yeast rice, niacin, fiber, soy protein

Other Natural Treatments
Indian mukul myrrh tree (guggulsterone), pantethine, L-carnitine, aortic glycosaminoglycans, chromium, calcium, multivitamin/mineral, lifestyle changes

One of the most significant discoveries in preventive medicine is that elevated levels of cholesterol in the blood accelerate atherosclerosis, or hardening of the arteries (see the discussion about cholesterol under Atherosclerosis). Along with high blood pressure, inactivity, smoking, and diabetes, high cholesterol has proven to be one of the most important promoters of heart disease, strokes, and peripheral vascular disease (blockage of circulation to the extremities, usually the legs).

Cholesterol does not directly clog arteries like grease clogs pipes. The current theory is that elevated levels of cholesterol irritate the walls of blood vessels and cause them to undergo harmful changes. Because most cholesterol is manufactured by the body itself, dietary sources of cholesterol (such as eggs) are not usually the most important problem. The relative proportion of unsaturated fats (from plants) and saturated fats (mainly from animal products) in the diet is more significant. The former lower cholesterol levels, whereas the latter raise them.

There is no question that increasing exercise and improving diet are the most important steps to take when cholesterol is high. These fundamental lifestyle changes are frequently effective and produce many benefits that go beyond simply lowering cholesterol levels.

However, if your cholesterol remains high despite your best efforts, you may need specific cholesterol-lowering treatments. There are a variety of effective drugs to choose from, and some, such as Pravachol (pravastatin), have actually been shown to prevent heart attacks and reduce mortality. While there are known and suspected risks associated with these medications, the benefits of these medications undoubtedly exceed the risks for those with significantly elevated cholesterol levels. In milder cases, however, some of the options described below might be better first choices.

Principal Natural Treatments for High Cholesterol

There are several herbs and supplements that can almost certainly help you lower your cholesterol level. However, before trying them, consult with your physician to find out whether you have time to experiment. If your cholesterol levels are very high and your arteries are already in bad condition, it might be wiser to turn to proven drug treatments. However, if your physician says that you can safely spend some time exploring your options, the treatments described in this section may be worth trying. (For more information, see *The Natural Pharmacist Guide to Garlic and Cholesterol*.)

Garlic: Strong Evidence It Reduces Total Cholesterol

The most well established herbal treatment for high cholesterol is the kitchen herb garlic. As far back as the first century A.D., Dioscorides wrote of garlic's ability to "clear the arteries." Today, Germany's Commission E authorizes the use of garlic "as an adjunct to dietary measures in patients with elevated blood lipids (cholesterol) and for the prevention of age-related vascular (blood vessel) changes."

The effectiveness of garlic appears to depend heavily on the formulation used. A relatively odorless substance, alliin, is one of the most important compounds in garlic and is believed by many researchers to be a prime active ingredient (or, technically, source of active ingredients). When garlic is crushed or cut, an enzyme called allinase is brought into contact with alliin, turning the latter into allicin. Allicin is most responsible for garlic's strong odor and may also play a major role in lowering cholesterol. The allicin itself then rapidly breaks down into entirely different compounds.

When you powder garlic to put it into a capsule, it acts like cutting the bulb. The chain reaction starts: Alliin contacts allinase, yielding allicin, which then breaks down.

Unless something is done to prevent this process, garlic powder will not have any alliin that can be turned into allicin left by the time you buy it.

Some garlic producers declare that alliin and allicin have nothing to do with garlic's effectiveness and simply sell products without either one, such as aged powdered garlic and garlic oil. However, there are serious doubts about the effectiveness of these products. Garlic oil, in particular, seems to be entirely ineffective (see What Is the Scientific Evidence for Garlic?).

Raw garlic is the most reliable source of alliin, but its strong odor keeps many people from using it. To solve this problem, manufacturers have devised ways to produce relatively odor-free garlic that still contains a standardized level of alliin. These are sold as powdered garlic with a guaranteed alliin content and, often, an "allicin potential" or "allicin yield."

What Is the Scientific Evidence for Garlic?

One of the best studies of garlic standardized to alliin content was conducted in Germany and published in 1990.[1] A total of 261 patients at 30 medical centers were given either 800 mg daily of garlic standardized to alliin content or placebo. Over the course of 16 weeks, patients in the treated group experienced a 12% drop in total cholesterol and a 17% decrease in triglyceride levels. The greatest benefits occurred in patients with initial cholesterol levels of 250 to 300 mg/dL.

All together, at least 28 controlled clinical studies have evaluated the effectiveness of garlic in lowering elevated cholesterol. Although some of these studies have shown no benefit even with standardized garlic,[2,3] overall the results make a reasonably good case that garlic powder standardized to alliin content can lower total cholesterol by about 9 to 12%.[4,5] We know much less about garlic's effects on LDL ("bad") cholesterol and HDL ("good") cholesterol.

There is also some evidence that aged garlic powder (without alliin) can lower cholesterol levels too, although perhaps to a lesser extent.[6] However, garlic oil appears to be ineffective.[7]

Garlic also appears to modestly reduce blood pressure (see the discussion of garlic under Hypertension). Furthermore, evidence suggests that it may soften artery walls through mechanisms other than lowering cholesterol and blood pressure,[8] perhaps by protecting against free radicals and hindering blood clotting.[9–16] Because of this multifaceted effect, many European physicians regard garlic as one of the best all-around treatments for the prevention of heart disease.

Dosage

In most of the studies that demonstrated the cholesterol-lowering powers of garlic, the daily dosage supplied at least 10 mg of alliin. This is sometimes stated in terms of how much allicin will be created from that alliin. The number you should look for is 4 to 5 mg of "allicin potential." You must allow at least 1 to 4 months of treatment for full effects.

Aged garlic without alliin may also offer some benefit, but don't bother with garlic oil.

Safety Issues

As a commonly used food, garlic is on the FDA's "generally regarded as safe" (GRAS) list. Rats have been fed gigantic doses of aged garlic (2,000 mg per kilogram body weight) for 6 months without any signs of negative effects.[17] Unfortunately, there is no safety information from animal studies on garlic powder standardized to alliin content, which is by far the most commonly used form of garlic.

The only common side effect of garlic is unpleasant breath odor. Even so-called odorless garlic produces an offensive smell in up to 50% of those who use it.[18]

Other side effects occur only rarely. For example, a study that followed 1,997 people who were given a normal dose of deodorized garlic daily over a 16-week period showed a 6% incidence of nausea, a 1.3% incidence of dizziness on standing (perhaps a sign of low blood pressure), and a 1.1% incidence of allergic reactions.[19] A few reports of bloating, headaches, sweating, and dizziness were also noted.

Raw garlic taken in excessive doses can cause many symptoms, including stomach upset, heartburn, nausea and vomiting, diarrhea, flatulence, facial flushing, rapid pulse, and insomnia.

Because garlic appears to possess blood-thinning effects, it might not be safe to combine garlic with blood thinners, such as Coumadin (warfarin), Trental (pentoxifylline), or aspirin, as well as other natural blood-thinning substances like ginkgo and vitamin E. High doses of garlic should not be taken before surgery or labor and delivery.

Maximum safe doses in young children, pregnant or nursing women, and those with severe kidney or liver disease has not been established. (For more information on garlic, see *The Natural Pharmacist Guide to Garlic and Cholesterol.*)

Red Yeast Rice: May Be Similar to Standard Drugs

Red yeast rice has recently arrived on the market as a treatment for lowering cholesterol. However, because of potential risks, it should only be used under physician supervision.

Red yeast rice is a traditional Chinese substance that is made by fermenting a type of yeast called *Monascus purpureus* over rice. This product (called Hong Qu) has been used in China since at least 800 A.D. as a food and also as a medicinal substance. Recently, it has been discovered that this ancient Chinese preparation contains at least 11 naturally occurring substances similar to prescription drugs in the "statin" family, such as Mevacor and Pravachol.

What Is the Scientific Evidence for Red Yeast Rice?

A double-blind placebo-controlled study followed 83 individuals given either 2,400 mg of red yeast rice daily or placebo for a period of 12 weeks.[20] The results showed an 18% drop in cholesterol in the treated group.

Most of the remaining research has been performed in China, and is not available in English form. Reportedly, over 15 controlled studies have been performed, showing that blood cholesterol may be reduced 11 to 32% with this product. Additional research is under way in the United States at the present time.

Dosage

For appropriate dosage, please refer to the labeling on the product.

Safety Issues

While there have been no serious adverse reactions reported in the studies of red yeast rice, some minor side effects have been reported. In the large study of 446 people, heartburn (1.8%), bloating (0.9%), and dizziness (0.3%) were all mentioned. Formal toxicity studies in rats and mice, giving doses up to 125 times the normal human dose for 3 months showed no toxic effects, according to unpublished information on file with one of the manufacturers of red rice yeast.[21]

However, because red yeast contains ingredients similar to the statin drugs, there is a theoretical risk of the same side effects and risks that are seen with those drugs. These include elevated liver enzymes, damage to skeletal muscle, and increase risk of cancer. Also, red yeast rice should not be combined with niacin, erythromycin, cyclosporine, other statin drugs, or the class of drugs called "fibrates." Serious side effects have occurred when statin drugs were combined with these medications.

This product should not be used by pregnant or nursing mothers or those with severe liver or kidney disease except on a physician's advice.

Niacin: A Treatment Accepted by Conventional Medicine

The common vitamin niacin is an accepted medical treatment for elevated cholesterol with solid science behind it. Unfortunately, niacin, if taken in sufficient quantities to lower cholesterol, can cause an annoying flushing reaction and occasionally liver inflammation.[22] It may also worsen blood sugar levels in people with diabetes. Close medical supervision is essential when using niacin to lower cholesterol.

To partially counter these problems, a special form of niacin has been developed in Europe: inositol hexaniacinate, or "flushless" niacin.[23] The term *flushless* is not quite accurate—some people do flush with inositol hexaniacinate, but the flush is neither as common nor as severe as with ordinary niacin. It is still necessary to check the liver periodically, so a physician's supervision remains essential.

The proper dosage of inositol hexaniacinate is 500 to 1,000 mg 3 times daily, taken with food. The usual recommendation is to start with the lower dose and raise it only if the cholesterol doesn't fall sufficiently after about 6 weeks.

Ordinary niacin can be used as well, and there are slow-release forms of niacin available by prescription. However, liver inflammation is a real possibility with all forms of niacin.

Fiber: Considered "Heart-Healthy" by the FDA

Water-soluble fiber supplements appear to lower cholesterol, and the FDA has permitted products containing this form of fiber to carry a "heart-healthy" label.[24] Many forms are available, ranging from oat bran to expensive fiber products sold through multilevel marketing firms. A good dose of oat bran is 5 to 10 g with each meal and at bedtime, and a good dose of psyllium is 10 g with each meal. However, eating a diet high in fresh fruits and vegetables and whole grains may be even better because of the many healthful nutrients such a diet contains.

Soy Protein: Soon to Be Labeled "Heart-Healthy"

Soy protein appears to lower total cholesterol by about 9%, LDL ("bad") cholesterol by 13%, and triglycerides by 10%.[25] At the time of this writing the FDA has proposed allowing foods containing soy protein to make this claim on the label. According to the FDA, it takes about 25 g of soy protein a day to get cholesterol-lowering effects. This amount can be found in H pound of tofu or 2H cups of soy milk.

Soy may not be safe for women with a previous history of breast cancer.

Other Natural Treatments for High Cholesterol

There are also several other promising alternative treatments for high cholesterol. Although the scientific evidence behind them is not yet strong, many alternative practitioners consider them to be highly effective.

A few preliminary double-blind studies suggest that an extract of the Indian mukul myrrh tree, known as gugulipid, may reduce total cholesterol about as effectively as garlic.[26,27,28] The dosage of standardized guggul should supply 25 mg of guggulsterone 3 times daily. Although side effects appear to be rare, detailed safety studies have not been performed; and safety in young children, pregnant or nursing women, and those with severe kidney or liver disease has not been established.

A special form of the vitamin pantothenic acid, known as pantethine, may significantly lower total blood triglycerides as well as cholesterol.[29,30,31] However, further research is necessary to prove the safety and effectiveness of this expensive supplement.

L-carnitine is another expensive supplement that may be able to improve cholesterol levels.[32] A typical dosage is 500 to 1,000 mg 3 times daily (for more information on L-carnitine, see the discussion under Angina).

Preliminary studies suggest that an extract from the lining of the aortas of cows, known as aortic glycosaminoglycans (GAGs), can improve cholesterol levels.[33,34,35] The typical dosage is 50 mg 2 times daily. Aortic GAGs are considered safe, as similar substances are widely found in foods.

Supplemental chromium may improve blood cholesterol in some people but not in others.[36] A typical safe dosage is 200 to 600 mcg of chromium picolinate daily. Calcium supplements may occasionally lower cholesterol.[37] A typical nutritional dosage is 500 to 1,000 mg daily.

Finally, because general nutrient deficiencies can alter cholesterol levels, a basic multivitamin and mineral may be useful.

Lifestyle Approaches

The dietary influence on cholesterol levels is enormous but not entirely understood. Clearly, saturated fats from animal sources raise cholesterol levels, whereas polyunsaturated fats (from plants) lower them.

Much discussion has taken place over precisely which types of nonanimal fats are best. Some studies point toward monounsaturated fats, such as those found in olive oil. Margarine, long thought to be "better than butter," now appears to be generally unhealthful. The hydrogenated or partially hydrogenated oils that make up margarine are found in other foods as well. However, at the time of this writing a special form of margarine from Finland is touted as being heart-healthy.

This is a rapidly evolving field, and anything I write here may be outdated by the time you read this. Consult a qualified health professional for the latest information.

Some observational studies have found an association between coffee intake and elevated cholesterol. However, because coffee use is typically associated with other bad habits, such as smoking and a diet high in animal fat, it is difficult to know for sure whether coffee is really causing the problem.[38]

Finally, other treatments that may help prevent or reverse atherosclerosis should be considered as well (see the discussion under Atherosclerosis).

COLDS AND FLUS

Principal Natural Treatments
Echinacea, andrographis, zinc, vitamin C, ginseng
Other Natural Treatments
Vitamin E, elderberry, ashwaganda, astragalus, garlic, suma, reishi, maitake, osha, yarrow, kudzu, ginger

A cold is a respiratory infection caused by one of hundreds of possible viruses. However, because these viruses are so widespread, it is perhaps more accurate to say that colds are caused by a decrease in immunity that allows one of these viruses to take hold.

Colds occur more frequently in winter, but no one knows exactly why. Nearly everyone catches colds occasionally; but some people catch colds quite frequently, and others tend to stay sick an unusually long time.

Conventional medicine can neither treat nor prevent the common cold. Furthermore, none of the over-the-counter treatments can shorten a cold, prevent complications such as sinus infections, or even provide significant temporary relief.

People often want to take antibiotics for colds, and many physicians will prescribe them—even though antibiotics have no effect on viruses. Many believe that when the mucus turns yellow, it means that a bacterial infection has occurred for which antibiotic treatment is indicated. However, viruses can also produce yellow mucus; and even if bacteria have made a home in the excess mucus, they may be only innocent bystanders and produce no symptoms.

Colds, however, can be complicated by bacterial infections. In such cases antibiotic treatment may be indicated. Decongestants and other symptomatic treatments have not been shown to be dramatically effective.

Principal Natural Treatments for Colds and Flus

Remember the old saying "a cold lasts seven days, but if you treat it properly you will get over it in a week"? Actually, it may be possible to do better than this by using the right natural supplement. A significant body of research suggests that the herb echinacea can significantly shorten colds and make them less severe. The herb andrographis and the nutritional supplements zinc and vitamin C also seem to help. However, we also don't know whether combining more than one of these treatments will produce better results.

While these treatments can help you get over a cold faster, there is little evidence that they prevent colds very well, if at all. However, there is one treatment that may actually prevent colds: the herb ginseng.

Echinacea: Reduces Cold and
Flu Symptoms and Helps Recovery

Until the 1930s, echinacea was the number-one cold and flu remedy in the United States. It lost its popularity with the arrival of sulfa antibiotics. Ironically, sulfa antibiotics are as ineffective against colds as any other antibiotic, while echinacea does seem to be at least somewhat helpful. In Germany, echinacea remains the main remedy for minor respiratory infections.

This herb is thought to be an immune stimulant, a type of treatment not found in conventional medicine. Drugs attack infections, but echinacea appears to activate the body's infection-fighting capacity. However, there is no evidence that echinacea strengthens or "nourishes" the immune system. It seems to just stimulate it into action.

There are three main species of echinacea: *Echinacea purpurea, Echinacea angustifolia,* and *Echinacea pallida. E. purpurea* is the most widely used, but the other two are also available. It isn't clear if any one type is better than the others. (For information on echinacea, see *The Natural Pharmacist Guide to Echinacea and Immunity*.)

What Is the Scientific Evidence for Echinacea?

An increasingly strong body of evidence suggests that, when taken at the onset of a cold or flu, echinacea can help you get better faster and reduce your symptoms while you are sick. It doesn't seem to have much (if any) effect on preventing colds.

One double-blind study found that in people with flu-like illnesses echinacea can significantly reduce symptoms such as headache, lethargy, cough, and aching limbs.[1] This study followed 100 people who had just become sick. Half received a combination herb product containing *E. angustifolia*, the other half a placebo. The results showed that the echinacea group experienced significantly less intense symptoms than the placebo group.

Another double-blind study of echinacea found similar benefits in 180 people with flu-like illnesses, who were given either placebo or 450 mg or 900 mg of *E. purpurea* daily.[2] By about the third day, those participants receiving the higher dose of echinacea (900 mg) showed noticeable benefits in the severity of symptoms. There was no real benefit in the placebo or low-dose echinacea group.

Another double-blind placebo-controlled study using the *E. pallida* species found that treatment reduced the length of colds by about 30%.[3] This study followed 160 adults who had just "caught cold." The results showed that treatment reduced the length of illness from 13 days to about 9.5 days, compared to placebo (these were rather long colds!).

Can echinacea prevent colds? The answer is probably not very well, if at all. In one double-blind study, 120 people were given *E. purpurea* or a placebo as soon as they started showing signs of getting a cold.[4] The results over the 10-day study period showed that fewer people in the echinacea group felt that their initial symptoms actually developed into "real" colds. However, the difference was only 20%. Again, the greatest benefit was helping the cold go away faster. Among those who did come down with "real" colds, improvement in the symptoms started much sooner in the echinacea group (4 days instead of 8 days).

Three other studies involving a total of over 400 participants found that regular use of *E. purpurea* or *E. angustifolia* did not prevent colds very well, if at all.[5,6,7] The bottom line is that echinacea can be counted on to lessen cold symptoms and help you recover faster, but not to prevent colds altogether.

How does echinacea work? The answer is that we really don't know. Both test-tube and animal studies have shown that the constituents found in echinacea can increase antibody production, raise white blood cell counts and stimulate the activity of key white blood cells.[8–13] However, it is far from certain that these findings really mean much! Many other substances cause similar changes, including wheat, bamboo, rice, sugarcane, and chamomile, and none of these has ever been considered an immune stimulant.[14]

Dosage

The three species of echinacea are used interchangeably. The typical daily dosage of echinacea powdered extract is 300 mg 3 times daily. Alcohol tincture (1:5) is usually taken at a dosage of 3 to 4 ml 3 times daily, echinacea juice at 2 to 3 ml 3 times daily, and whole dried root at 1 to 2 g 3 times daily. Echinacea is usually taken at the first sign of a cold and continued for 7 to 14 days. Long-term use is probably not helpful.

There is no broad agreement on which ingredients should be standardized in echinacea tinctures and solid extracts. However, echinacea juice is often standardized to contain 2.4% of beta-1,2-fructofuranoside.

Many herbalists feel that liquid forms of echinacea are more effective than tablets or capsules because they believe that part of echinacea's benefit is due to direct contact with the tonsils and other lymphatic tissues at the back of the throat.[15] These tissues act as an early warning system for infections. By stimulating them, echinacea may encourage the body to fight a cold more promptly.

Finally, goldenseal is frequently combined with echinacea in cold preparations. However, there is no evidence that oral goldenseal stimulates immunity, nor did traditional herbalists use it for this purpose.[16] (For more information on goldenseal, see *The Natural Pharmacist: Your Complete Guide to Herbs.*)

Safety Issues

Echinacea appears to be very safe. Even when taken in very high doses, it does not appear to cause any toxic effects.[17,18] Side effects are also rare and usually limited to minor gastrointestinal symptoms, increased urination, and allergic reactions.[19]

Germany's Commission E warns against using echinacea if you have an autoimmune disorder such as multiple sclerosis, lupus, or rheumatoid arthritis, as well as tuberculosis or leukocytosis. Rumors say that echinacea should not be used if you have AIDS. These warnings are purely theoretical, being based on fears that echinacea might actually activate immunity in the wrong way. While no evidence shows that echinacea use has actually harmed anyone with these diseases, caution is advisable.

Germany's Commission E also recommends against using echinacea for more than 8 weeks. Since there is no evidence that echinacea is effective when taken long term, this is probably sensible. The safety of echinacea in pregnant or nursing women, and those with severe kidney or liver disease has not been established. In German studies from the 1950s and 60s, more than 1,000 children were given injected forms of echinacea, with no apparent harm.[20] Given these findings, it seems likely that oral echinacea is safe in children, but we don't know this for sure.

Andrographis: A Promising Treatment for Colds

Andrographis is a shrub found throughout India and other Asian countries, sometimes called "Indian echinacea" because it is believed to provide much the same benefits. It was widely used during the terrible influenza epidemics that occurred earlier this century. Recently, it has become popular in Scandinavia as a treatment for colds.

What Is the Scientific Evidence for Andrographis?

According to a few well-designed studies, andrographis can both reduce the symptoms and shorten the duration of colds.

In one double-blind study, 50 people with colds were given either andrographis or placebo.[21] Researchers reported that 55% of the treated participants reported that their colds were less intense than usual, while only 19% of those in the placebo group stated this. The treated group averaged only 0.2 days of sick leave, while the group taking placebo averaged 1 full day of sick leave. Finally, 75% of the treated participants were well after 5 days, compared to less than 40% in the placebo group.

Another double-blind study that enrolled 59 people concluded that andrographis could reduce cold symptoms such as fatigue, sore throat, sore muscles, runny nose, headache, and lymph node swelling.[22] Participants received either 1,200 mg of andrographis (standardized to 4% andrographolides) or a placebo. By the fourth day of the study, the andrographis group showed definite improvement in most of their cold symptoms as compared to the placebo group.

Finally, a double-blind study involving 152 adults compared the effectiveness of andrographis (at either 3 g per day or 6 g per day) versus acetaminophen for sore throat and fever.[23] The higher dose of andrographis (6 g) decreased symptoms of fever and throat pain, as did acetaminophen, while the lower dose of andrographis (3 g) did not. There were no significant side effects in either group.

These studies do not tell us whether andrographis improves immunity or simply relieves symptoms. Still, the results are quite promising and suggest that this herb deserves further study.

Dosage

A typical dosage of andrographis is a ½ to 1 teaspoon 3 times daily, taken with lots of liquids at mealtimes. Andrographis is typically standardized to its andrographolide content, usually 15 to 30% in many commercial products. However, the 59-person study described above used a product standardized to 4% andrographolides.

Safety Issues

No significant adverse effects have been reported in human studies of andrographis. The 59-person study mentioned earlier asked participants to report side effects, in addition to monitoring lab tests for liver function, complete blood counts, kidney function, and some other laboratory measures of toxicity.[24] All of their tests were within the normal limits for both the placebo and the andrographis groups.

However, full formal safety studies have not been completed. This means that the herb is not recommended for young children, pregnant or nursing women, or those with severe liver or kidney disease.

There are some concerns from animal studies that andrographis may impair fertility. One study showed that male rats became infertile when fed 20 mg of andrographis powder per day.[25] In this case, the rats stopped producing sperm and exhibited physical changes in some of the testicular cells involved in sperm production. Researchers also detected evidence of degeneration of structures in the testicles. However, another study showed no evidence of testicular toxicity in male rats that were given up to 1 g per kilogram of body weight per day for 60 days, so this issue remains unclear.[26]

One group of female mice also did not fare well on andrographis.[27] When fed 2 g per kilogram body weight daily for 6 weeks (thousands of times higher than the usual human dose), all female mice failed to get pregnant when mated with males of proven fertility. Meanwhile, of the control females, 95.2% got pregnant when mated with a similar group of male mice.

While andrographis is probably not a useful form of birth control, these animal studies are somewhat worrisome and warrant further investigation.

Zinc: Appears Effective, but Research Is Contradictory

Another famous alternative treatment for colds is the use of zinc lozenges. In cases of zinc deficiency, the immune system does not function properly.[28,29] Because zinc is commonly deficient in the diet, especially among senior citizens,[30] nutritional zinc supplementation may certainly be useful for those who get sick easily. Indeed, a recent 2-year, double-blind study suggests that zinc and selenium taken together in nutritional doses can reduce the number of infections in nursing home residents.[31]

However, zinc is most commonly recommended to be used in a different way: sucking on high doses of zinc lozenges at the onset of cold symptoms. This method may work by directly killing viruses in the throat rather than improving the nutritional status of the body.

What Is the Scientific Evidence for Zinc?

A recent double-blind study concluded that proper use of zinc lozenges can cause many cold symptoms to go away faster than they would otherwise.[32] In this trial, 100 people who were experiencing the early symptoms of a cold were given a lozenge that either contained 13.3 mg of zinc from zinc gluconate or was just a placebo. Participants took the lozenges several times daily until their cold symptoms subsided. The results were impressive. Coughing disappeared within 2.2 days in the treated group versus 4 days in the placebo group. Sore throat disappeared after 1 day versus

3 days in the placebo group, nasal drainage in 4 days (versus 7 days), and headache in 2 days (versus 3 days).

Not all studies have shown such positive results.[33] However, the overall results appear to be favorable.[34] It has been suggested that the exact formulation of the zinc lozenge plays a significant role. Sweetening agents, such as sorbitol, mannitol, and the flavorings citric acid and tartaric acid, appear to prevent zinc from killing viruses, and chemical forms of zinc other than zinc gluconate or zinc acetate may not work.[35]

However, one recent trial with exactly the right form of zinc lozenge found no benefit in children, for reasons that are not clear.[36] The bottom line is that while zinc probably does help in colds, more research is needed.

Dosage

The typical dosage is 23 mg of zinc gluconate, taken every 2 hours at the earliest signs of a cold and continued for no more than 1 week.

For long-term nutritional supplementation of zinc, 10 to 30 mg daily is generally recommended. Zinc can cause copper deficiency, so it should be combined with 1 to 3 mg of copper daily.

Safety Issues

The short-term use of zinc is believed to be safe. However, high doses of zinc should not be kept up for more than 1 week because such doses can actually depress the immune system and cause other symptoms if taken for too long. As mentioned previously, zinc can also deplete the body of copper.

Vitamin C: Not a Cure, but It Helps

Vitamin C is the most famous of all natural treatments for colds, and it has been subjected to irresponsible hype from both its proponents and opponents. However, if you take a fair look at the research record, it appears that vitamin C can significantly reduce symptoms of colds and help you get over your cold faster.[37,38]

In five studies, in which people took 70 to 200 mg of vitamin C daily, cold symptoms were decreased by about 30%. In 11 other studies that used a higher dosage (1,000 mg or more), symptoms were reduced by 40%.

However, vitamin C does not seem to prevent colds very well, except perhaps those connected with serious endurance exercise such as marathon running.[39,40,41]

A typical dosage is 500 to 1,000 mg 3 to 6 times daily while cold symptoms last. The short-term use of high doses of vitamin C is believed to be safe, although diarrhea may occur.

Ginseng: May Actually Prevent Colds

Although most people in the West think of ginseng as a stimulant, in Eastern Europe, ginseng is widely believed to improve overall immunity to illness. As we have seen, echinacea does not seem to prevent colds. But it appears that regular use of ginseng may be able to provide this important benefit.

There are actually three different herbs commonly called ginseng: Asian ginseng (*Panax ginseng*), American ginseng (*Panax quinquefolius*), and Siberian "ginseng" (*Eleutherococcus senticosus*). The latter herb is actually not ginseng at all, but some herbalists believe that it functions identically.

What Is the Scientific Evidence for Ginseng?

Unfortunately, most of the scientific studies on ginseng have involved animals who received ginseng injections straight into the abdomen. However, a recent, properly performed, double-blind placebo-controlled study looked at the potential immune-stimulating effects of *Panax ginseng* when taken by mouth.[42] This trial enrolled 227 individuals at three medical offices in Milan, Italy. Half were given ginseng at a dose of 100 mg daily, and the other half took placebo. Four weeks into the study, all participants received influenza vaccine.

The results showed a significant decline in the frequency of colds and flus in the treated group compared to the placebo group (15 versus 42 cases). Also, antibody measurements in response to the vaccination rose higher in the treated group than in the placebo group.

While more research is needed, this study suggests that ginseng may be able to do what echinacea, andrographis, zinc lozenges, and vitamin C cannot: prevent colds.

Dosage

The typical recommended daily dose of _Panax ginseng_ is 1 to 2 g of raw herb, or 200 mg daily of an extract standardized to contain 4 to 7% ginsenosides. _Eleutherococcus_ is taken at a dosage of 2 to 3 g whole herb or 300 to 400 mg of extract daily.

Ordinarily, a 2- to 3-week period of using ginseng is recommended, followed by a 1- to 2-week "rest" period. Russian tradition suggests that ginseng should not be used by those under 40 years old.

Safety Issues

The various forms of ginseng appear to be nontoxic, both in the short and long term, according to the results of studies in mice, rats, chickens, and dwarf pigs. Ginseng also does not seem to be carcinogenic.[43,44,45]

Side effects are rare. Occasionally women report menstrual abnormalities and/or breast tenderness when they take ginseng, and overstimulation and insomnia have also been reported. Unconfirmed reports suggest that highly excessive dosages of ginseng can raise blood pressure, increase heart rate, and possibly cause other significant effects. Whether some of these cases were actually caused by caffeine mixed in with ginseng remains unclear.

Ginseng allergy can also occur, as can allergy to any other substance.

In 1979, an article was published in the *Journal of the American Medical Association* claiming that people can become addicted to ginseng and develop blood pressure elevation, nervousness, sleeplessness, diarrhea, and hypersexuality. This report has since been thoroughly discredited and should no longer be taken seriously.[46,47]

However, an unpublished report suggests that ginseng can interfere with drug metabolism, specifically those processed by an enzyme called "CYP 3A4." Ask your physician or pharmacist whether you are taking any medications of this type. There have also been specific reports of ginseng interacting with MAO inhibitor drugs and digitalis, although again it is not clear whether it was the ginseng or a contaminant that caused the problem.

Safety in young children, pregnant or nursing women, or those with severe liver or kidney disease has not been established. Interestingly, Chinese tradition suggests that ginseng should not be used during pregnancy or lactation.

Other Natural Treatments for Colds and Flus

There is some evidence that vitamin E may improve immune function, but whether this translates into an effect on colds has not been determined.[48]

A recent study suggests that the herb elderberry can significantly reduce the length and severity of flu symptoms.[49] Elderberry-flower tea is made by steeping 3 to 5 g of dried flowers in one cup of boiling water for 10 to 15 minutes. A typical dosage is 1 cup 3 times daily. Standardized extracts should be taken according to the directions on the product's label.

Elderberry flower is generally regarded as safe. Side effects are rare and consist primarily of occasional mild gastrointestinal distress or allergic reactions. Nonetheless, safety in young children, pregnant or nursing women, or those with severe liver or kidney disease is not established.

Various other herbs are said to work like ginseng and enhance immunity over the long term, including ashwaganda, astragalus, garlic, suma, reishi, and maitake. However, there is no good evidence that they really work. Other herbs, including osha, yarrow, kudzu, and ginger, are said to help avert colds when taken at the first sign of infection; but again, there is no scientific evidence that they are effective.

CONGESTIVE HEART FAILURE

Principal Natural Treatments
Coenzyme Q$_{10}$, hawthorn
Other Natural Treatments
Taurine, L-carnitine, magnesium

When the heart sustains injury that weakens its pumping ability, a complicated physiological state called congestive heart failure (CHF) can develop. Fluid builds up in the lungs and lower extremities, the heart enlarges, and many symptoms develop, including severe fatigue, difficulty breathing while lying down, and altered brain function.

Medical treatment for this condition is quite effective and sophisticated and consists of several drugs used in combination.

Principal Natural Treatments for Congestive Heart Failure

CHF is too serious a condition for self-treatment. The supervision of a qualified health-care professional is essential. For this reason, I deliberately do not give detailed dosage information in this section. However, given medical supervision, some of the following treatments may be quite useful. In Japan and Europe, coenzyme Q_{10} is frequently added to standard treatment for added benefit. The herb hawthorn alone may be effective for mild CHF.

Coenzyme Q_{10}: Can Be Taken with Standard Medical Treatment

The substance known as coenzyme Q_{10} (CoQ_{10}) appears to be quite helpful when combined with standard treatment for CHF. CoQ_{10} occurs naturally in the energy-producing subunits of all plant and animal cells (the mitochondria). This safe supplement is widely used in Europe, Israel, and Japan as an approved treatment for a variety of cardiovascular conditions.

One double-blind study followed 80 people with CHF and found that adding CoQ_{10} to standard treatment significantly improved heart function.[1] Another study tracked 641 individuals for 1 full year and found both improved symptoms and a reduced need for hospitalization.[2] CoQ_{10} appears to be essentially nontoxic and side-effect free.[3]

(For more information on CoQ_{10}, see *The Natural Pharmacist: Your Complete Guide to Vitamins and Supplements*.)

Hawthorn: Approved in Germany for Mild CHF

The name hawthorn drives from "hedgethorn," reflecting this spiny tree's use as a living fence in much of Europe. During the Middle Ages, hawthorn was used to treat dropsy, a condition that we now call CHF. It was also used for other heart ailments and for sore throat.

Hawthorn is widely regarded in modern Europe as a safe and effective treatment for the early stages of CHF. Although not as potent as that other famous heart herb of the Middle Ages, foxglove (digitalis), hawthorn is much safer. The active ingredients in foxglove are the drugs digoxin and digitoxin. However, hawthorn does not appear to have any single active ingredient. This has prevented it from being turned into a drug.

Like digitalis, hawthorn speeds up the heart and increases its force of contraction. However, it may offer one very important advantage. Digitalis and other medications that increase the power of the heart also make it more irritable and liable to dangerous irregularities of rhythm. In contrast, hawthorn appears to have the unique property of both strengthening the heart and stabilizing it against arrythmias.[4,5,6] Also, with digitalis the difference between the proper dose and the toxic dose is very small. Hawthorn has an enormous range of safe dosing.[7]

Between 1981 and 1994, 13 controlled clinical studies of hawthorn were conducted, most of them double-blind.[8] A total of 808 people participated in these trials. The collective results strongly suggest that hawthorn is an effective treatment for early stages of CHF. Comparative studies suggest that hawthorn is about as effective as a low dose of the conventional drug captopril.

Note: Although captopril and other standard drugs in the same family have been shown to reduce mortality associated with CHF, there is no similar evidence for hawthorn.

Hawthorn appears to be quite safe. Germany's Commission E lists no known risks, contraindications, or drug interactions with hawthorn, and mice and rats have been given phenomenal doses without showing significant toxicity.[9] However, because hawthorn obviously affects the heart, it should not be combined with other heart drugs without a physician's supervision.

Side effects are also rare and consist mainly of mild stomach upset and occasional allergic reactions (skin rash). Safety in young children, pregnant or nursing women, and those with severe kidney or liver disease has not been established.

Other Natural Treatments
for Congestive Heart Failure

At least one double-blind study suggests that the amino acid taurine may be useful in CHF.[10,11] Taurine is believed to be safe.

Another treatment for CHF that has some evidence is the expensive supplement L-carnitine, especially when given in the special form called L-propionyl-carnitine.[12–15] (For more information about carnitine, see the discussion under Angina.) Carnitine is frequently combined with CoQ_{10}.

There is also some evidence that supplementing with magnesium may be useful.

Finally, it is important to pay attention to all the general considerations that bring health to the heart, such as those described in Atherosclerosis.

CONSTIPATION

Principal Natural Treatments
Increased dietary fiber (psyllium husks, debittered fenugreek seeds, and flaxseed) and water intake, *Cascara sagrada*

In the nineteenth century, a naturopathic concept came into being whose influence persists today: namely, that regular, frequent, and complete bowel movements are necessary for optimum health. William Harvey Kellogg, of Kellogg's cereal fame, wrote extensively of the dangers of "auto-intoxication" purportedly caused by inadequate elimination. He and others claimed that a concrete-like sludge builds up on the wall of the colon, increasing in thickness over time and destroying the health of the body.

However, in modern times physicians have performed millions of direct examinations of the colon, using the procedure known as colonoscopy, without finding any evidence of such a coating. Caked colons are a myth.

Furthermore, conventional medicine has never observed any connection between elimination and overall health. Many people eliminate only once a week or so, and their health appears to be no worse than that of the population at large. Nonetheless, most people find constipation unpleasant, and for some it becomes a severe chronic problem.

Conventional treatment for constipation involves mainly increasing exercise and intake of dietary fiber and water while reserving laxatives, suppositories, and enemas for emergencies.

Principal Natural Treatments for Constipation

Occasional constipation can be safely self-treated. However, if constipation becomes a chronic problem, it should be evaluated by a physician.

Increasing dietary fiber and water intake is the first treatment to try for chronic constipation. Some of the most useful forms of fiber are psyllium husks, debittered fenugreek seeds, and flaxseed. A typical dosage is 5 to 10 g 1 to 3 times daily, with at least 16 ounces of liquid. Start with the lower doses and work up gradually, as too much fiber all at once can actually worsen constipation.

The herb *Cascara sagrada* is an approved over-the-counter treatment for constipation. However, when taken by itself, it can occasionally cause dependence. It is often combined in small amounts with other herbs, including barberry, turkey rhubarb, red raspberry, goldenseal, and cayenne, that gently affect the digestive tract. However, the safety and efficacy of these combinations have not been proven.

A final point about constipation: Like sleep, elimination is inhibited by thinking too much about it. Part of the key to solving chronic constipation problems is to decrease the sense of worry and anxiety that surround the issue. Although constipation is certainly unpleasant, its evils have been greatly exaggerated. Thinking less about it will often go a long way toward solving the problem.

CYCLIC MASTALGIA
(Cyclic Mastitis, Fibrocystic Breast Disease)

Principal Natural Treatments
Evening primrose oil, ginkgo, chasteberry

Some women's breasts are unusually tender and lumpy, with symptoms of pain and dull heaviness that vary with the menstrual cycle. This condition is called cyclic mastalgia or mastitis and is often associated with premenstrual stress syndrome (PMS). When the lumps become significant enough to be called cysts, this condition is sometimes called fibrocystic breast disease.

Besides discomfort, perhaps the worst problem of this condition is that it can mimic the appearance of breast cancer on mammograms, leading to false alarms. To make matters worse, fibrocystic changes can also hide true cancers, and women with fibrocystic breast disease may also have a greater tendency toward breast cancer (although this is controversial).

Conventional treatment of cyclic mastalgia has incorporated many staples of alternative medicine. After screening carefully for breast cancer, physicians typically recommend reducing animal fats, avoiding chocolate and caffeine, and supplementing with vitamin E (400 IU daily) and vitamin B_6 (50 mg daily). Some physicians have begun to use evening primrose oil as well. These treatments are more likely to be successful in cases that involve pain but no cysts. Even so, the response to therapy is slow, often requiring over 6 months for full results.

If these natural methods don't work, physicians may prescribe various hormone or hormone-like medications.

Principal Natural Treatments for Cyclic Mastalgia

Cyclic mastalgia often occurs in connection with PMS. (See PMS for information on related treatments.)

Evening Primrose Oil

European physicians commonly use evening primrose oil (EPO) to treat cyclic mastalgia, and the practice has come to be popular among some physicians in the United States as well. EPO contains relatively high concentrations of the essential fatty acid gamma-linolenic acid (GLA). Fatty acid metabolism is known to be disturbed in women with cyclic mastalgia, and abnormalities in essential fatty acid levels have been found in women with PMS and with non-malignant breast disease.[1] It appears that supplementation with EPO may be able to correct this imbalance.

What Is the Scientific Evidence for EPO?

In uncontrolled studies, EPO has been found to produce significant benefits in about 44% of women with cyclic mastalgia.[2]

Improvement was also seen in a controlled study of 73 women suffering from cyclic breast pain.[3] Discomfort was significantly reduced in the group taking EPO, whereas no significant improvement was seen in the placebo group.

However, EPO does not seem to be helpful when there are breast cysts rather than just pain. In a 1-year double-blind study of 200 women with breast cysts, EPO did not prove effective.[4,5]

Dosage

A typical dosage of EPO is 2 to 3 g daily. It must be taken for at least 4 to 6 weeks for noticeable effect, and maximum benefits may require 4 to 8 months to develop. Borage oil and black currant oil contain similar ingredients and are sometimes used instead (see Safety Issues).

Safety Issues

EPO appears to be safe. (For more information on EPO, see Essential Fatty Acids under Diabetes.) There are concerns that certain preparations of borage oil may contain substances that could be toxic to the liver.

Ginkgo

Although the herb ginkgo is primarily used to enhance memory and mental function (see Alzheimer's Disease), it may be helpful for breast tenderness as well. A double-blind study evaluated 143 women with PMS symptoms, 18 to 45 years of age, and followed them for two menstrual cycles.[6] When the study began, each woman received either the ginkgo extract or placebo on day 16 of the first cycle. Treatment was continued until day 5 of the next cycle, and resumed again on the day 16 of that cycle.

The results were impressive. As compared to placebo, ginkgo significantly relieved major symptoms of PMS, especially breast pain.

Dosage

The form of ginkgo used in the study I just described and in all other scientific trials is a highly concentrated extract, in which 50 pounds of the leaf must be used to create 1 pound of product. Such extracts are standardized to contain 24% by weight substances known as ginkgo flavonol glycosides. The proper dosage of ginkgo is 40 to 80 mg 3 times daily. It should be taken from about 2 weeks prior to your menstrual period until bleeding stops.

Safety Issues

Ginkgo extract appears to be quite safe. A review of nearly 10,000 participants taking ginkgo extract showed that less than 1% experienced side effects, and those that did occur were minor.[7] In another study, overall side effects were no greater in the ginkgo group than in the placebo group.[8] When a medication produces no more side effects than the placebo, we can reasonably regard it as essentially side-effect free. Furthermore, according to animal studies, ginkgo is safe even when taken in massive overdose.[9]

However, taking ginkgo presents one potential concern. The herb possesses a mild blood-thinning effect that could conceivably cause bleeding problems in certain situations. For this reason, people with hemophilia should not take ginkgo except on a physician's advice. Using ginkgo in the weeks prior to or just after major surgery or labor and delivery is also not advisable. Finally, ginkgo should not be combined with blood-thinning drugs such as Coumadin (warfarin), heparin, aspirin, and Trental (pentoxifylline) except under medical supervision. Ginkgo might also conceivably interact with natural products that slightly thin the blood as well, such as garlic and high-dose vitamin E.

The safety of ginkgo for young children, pregnant or nursing women, and people with kidney or liver disease has not been established.

Chasteberry

In Germany, the herb chasteberry is frequently used to treat cyclic mastalgia and other symptoms of PMS.[10,11,12] (For a detailed discussion of chasteberry use and safety issues, see PMS.)

DEPRESSION
(Mild to Moderate)

Principal Natural Treatments

St. John's wort

Other Natural Treatments

Phenylalanine, 5-hydroxytryptophan, ginkgo, phosphatidylserine, S-adenosylmethionine, inositol, vitamin B_6, vitamin B_{12}, folic acid

Not Recommended Treatments

Yohimbe, DHEA

Depression is a common emotional illness that varies widely in its intensity from person to person. The natural treatments described in this section are useful only for mild to moderate depressive symptoms consisting mainly of depressed mood, fatigue, insomnia, irritability, and difficulty concentrating.

More severe depression includes severely depressed mood complicated by symptoms such as slowed speech, slowed (or agitated) responses, markedly impaired memory and concentration, excessive (or diminished) sleep, significant weight loss (or weight gain), intense feelings of worthlessness and guilt, recurrent thoughts of suicide, and lack of interest in pleasurable activities.

Severe clinical depression is a dangerous and excruciating illness. The emotional structure of the brain has frozen into a pattern of misery that cannot be altered by willpower, a change of scenery, or the most earnest efforts of friends. In a sense, the brain has locked up like a crashed computer. No alternative treatment is especially successful when depression gets this bad.

One of the earliest successful treatments for major depression was shock therapy. This technique is almost the exact equivalent of rebooting a computer, and in cases of major depression its effects were revolutionary. For the first time, a reliable way was available to bring people out of the depths of severe major depression. However, shock treatment was overused at first and became unpopular.

The accidental discovery of antidepressant drugs provided a less interventive route. The original antidepressants, known as MAO inhibitors, could bring people out from the depths of major depression as successfully as shock treatment. However, MAO inhibitors can cause serious and even fatal side effects. No one would ever think of using MAO inhibitors to treat mild to moderate depression.

Subsequently, antidepressants with progressively fewer side effects came on the market, but it was not until the appearance of selective serotonin-reuptake inhibitors (SSRIs), such as Prozac and related drugs, that antidepressants became a viable option for depression that was less than catastrophic. Practically overnight, enormous numbers of people began taking Prozac and similar antidepressants for mild to moderate depression.

The big advantage of the SSRIs is that they don't cause fatigue. Many people find them to be entirely side-effect free. However, side effects are not uncommon, and include nausea, insomnia, and sexual disturbances (such as the loss of the ability to experience an orgasm).

Principal Natural Treatments for Depression

Alternative medicine offers one solidly proven treatment for depression: the herb St. John's wort. The evidence for this herb's effectiveness is nearly as comprehensive as what is required of a drug prior to approval. However, St. John's wort is only useful for mild to moderate depression. For severe depression, conventional antidepressant drugs are necessary and may be lifesaving.

St. John's Wort: A Well-Established
Treatment for Mild to Moderate Depression

St. John's wort (*Hypericum perforatum*) is a common perennial herb, with many branches and bright yellow flowers, that grows wild in much of the world. Its name derives from the herb's tendency to flower around the feast of St. John (wort simply means "plant" in Old English). The species name *perforatum* derives from the water-marking of translucent dots that can be seen when a leaf of the plant is held up to the sun.

St. John's wort has a long history of use in emotional disorders. It began to be considered as a treatment for depression early in the twentieth century, and when pharmaceutical antidepressants were invented, German researchers looked for similar properties in St. John's wort.

Today, St. John's wort is one of the best-documented herbal treatments, with a scientific record approaching that of many prescription drugs. Indeed, this herb is a prescription antidepressant in Germany. It is covered by that country's national health-care system and is prescribed more frequently than any synthetic drug. At the time of this writing, St. John's wort has also become the most commonly used antidepressant in the United States.

St. John's wort is used for mild to moderate depression. Typical symptoms include depressed mood, lack of energy, sleep problems, anxiety, appetite disturbance, difficulty concentrating, and poor stress tolerance. Irritability can also be a sign of depression.

St. John's wort appears to be effective in about 55% of cases. As with other antidepressants, the full benefit takes about 4 to 6 weeks to develop. The most common reported effects are brightened mood, increased energy, and improved sleep.

The big advantage of St. John's wort over standard medications is that it rarely, if ever, causes side effects.

However, St. John's wort should never be relied on to treat severe depression. If you or a loved one are feeling suicidal, unable to cope with daily life, paralyzed by anxiety, incapable of getting out of bed, unable to sleep, or uninterested in eating, see a physician at once. Drug therapy may save your life.

Like other antidepressants, St. John's wort can also be used to treat chronic insomnia and anxiety when they are related to depression. It may be effective in seasonal affective disorder (SAD) as well.

What Is the Scientific Evidence for St. John's Wort?

All together, at least 15 double-blind studies comparing St. John's wort to placebo have been reported at the time of this writing.[1,2] A review that evaluated most of these studies found that nine of them were performed according to adequate scientific standards, involving a total of over 600 participants.[3] According to the review author, "on the basis of the published, scientifically compelling evidence, Hypericum represents an effective therapy for the alleviation of the symptoms of depression." This body of research has been criticized by some authorities who point out that none of the studies exceeded 8 weeks in length. However, as it states in the *Physicians' Desk Reference,* Prozac was approved on the basis of studies that lasted no longer than 6 weeks.

How Does St. John's Wort Work?

We do not really know how St. John's wort acts. Early research suggested that it works like the oldest class of antidepressants, the MAO inhibitors.[4] However, later research essentially discredited this idea.[5,6] More recent research has focused on a connection between St. John's wort and serotonin.[7,8] The substance hyperforin may be a major active ingredient in St. John's wort.[9]

Dosage

The standard dosage of St. John's wort is 300 mg 3 times daily of an extract standardized to contain 0.3% hypericin. Recently, a new form of the herb has come on the market standardized to 3 to 5% hyperforin instead. However, the dosage amount is the same. Some people take 600 mg of St. John's wort in the morning and 300 mg at night, or some other variation on the same total daily dose. This dosage should not be exceeded, as it is not clear that higher doses produce any better effects, and the chance of side effects might increase.

If the herb bothers your stomach, take it with food. Remember that the full effect takes 4 weeks to develop, so don't give up too soon!

Warning: Various systemic diseases, such as hypothyroidism, chronic hepatitis, and anemia, may masquerade as depression. Make sure to find out whether you have an undiagnosed medical illness before treating yourself with St. John's wort.

Also, it can sometimes be difficult to assess the true intensity of your own depression. A physician's evaluation is essential. If you suffer from severe major depression, you should take medications rather than St. John's wort.

Safety Issues

St. John's wort is essentially side-effect free. Strangely, this good news has an unfortunate consequence: Some people who try St. John's wort decide that it must not be very powerful because it doesn't make them feel ill, so they quit. Be patient!

In a study designed to look for side effects, 3,250 people took St. John's wort for 4 weeks.[10] Overall, about 2.4% experienced side effects. The most common were mild stomach discomfort (0.6%), allergic reactions, mainly rash (0.5%), tiredness (0.4%), and restlessness (0.3%).

In the extensive German experience with St. John's wort as a treatment for depression, no reports of serious adverse consequences or drug interactions have been published.[11] Animal studies involving enormous doses for 26 weeks have not shown any serious toxicity.[12]

Cows and sheep grazing on St. John's wort have sometimes developed severe and even fatal sensitivity to the sun. However, this has never occurred in humans taking St. John's wort at normal doses.[13] In one study, highly sunsensitive people were given twice the normal dose of the herb.[14] The results showed a mild but measurable increase in reaction to ultraviolet radiation. The moral of the story is that if you are especially sensitive to the sun, do not exceed the recommended dosage of St. John's wort and continue to take your usual precautions against burning.

Older reports suggested that St. John's wort works like the class of drugs known as MAO inhibitors.[15] This led to a number of warnings, including avoiding cheese and decongestants while taking St. John's wort. However, this concern is no longer considered realistic.[16,17]

Safety in young children, pregnant or nursing women, and those with severe liver or kidney disease has not been established.

Drug Interactions

Some authorities suggest that combining St. John's wort with drugs in the Prozac family (SSRIs) might raise serotonin too much and cause a number of serious problems. Although there are as yet no official reports of such interactions (at the time of this writing) doctors have begun to informally report cases of this so-called serotonin syndrome. I recommend that you do not combine St. John's wort with prescription antidepressants.

An additional wrinkle to consider is that some drugs, such as Prozac, can take a long time to wash out of your system. If you stop Prozac, you may need to wait 3 weeks or more before starting St. John's wort.

It has been recently reported that St. John's wort lowers blood levels of theophylline, an asthma medication. Unpublished data from the University of Colorado suggest that the hypericin in St. John's wort may increase the activity of an enzyme called cytochrome P-450.[18,19] This substance is responsible for metabolizing many drugs and other chemicals. By increasing P-450 activity, St. John's wort may cause the body to break down these drugs faster, thereby making them less effective. Before taking St. John's wort, it might be a good idea to ask your physician whether any of your medications would be affected by "cytochrome P-450 CYP 1A1 and 1A2 induction."

Another study out of the University of Colorado suggests that St. John's wort may interfere with the action of the antitumor drugs etoposide (VePesid), teniposide (Vumon), mitoxantrone (Novantrone), and doxorubicin (Adriamycin).[20]

Other Natural Treatments for Depression

There are a number of other herbs and supplements that may be helpful in depression, although the evidence for them is not as strong as that for St. John's wort.

Phenylalanine: A Promising Treatment for Depression

Phenylalanine is a naturally occurring amino acid that we all consume in our daily diets. There is some evidence that phenylalanine supplements may help reduce symptoms of depression.

What Is the Scientific Evidence for Phenylalanine?

Phenylalanine occurs in a right-hand and a left-hand form, known as D- and L-phenylalanine, respectively. Some studies have evaluated the D form and others the L form, and still others have evaluated mixtures of both. All forms seem to be able to provide some measure of relief for symptoms of depression. The mixed form (DLPA) is the form most commonly available in stores.

A 1978 study compared the effectiveness of D-phenylalanine against the antidepressant drug imipramine (taken in daily doses of 100 mg) and found them to be equally effective.[21] A total of 60 individuals were randomly assigned to either one group or the other and followed for 30 days. D-phenylalanine worked more rapidly, producing significant improvement in only 15 days.

Another double-blind study followed 27 people, half of whom received DL-phenylalanine and the other half imipramine in higher doses of 150 to 200 mg daily.[22,23] When the participants were reevaluated in 30 days, the two groups had improved by the same amount.

Unfortunately, there do not seem to have been any properly designed studies that compared phenylalanine to placebo. Until these are performed, phenylalanine cannot be considered a proven treatment for depression, but it is certainly promising.

Dosage

A typical dosage is 150 to 400 mg of DL-phenylalanine daily, divided into 2 or 3 doses.

Safety Issues

There are few reported side effects with phenylalanine, although increased anxiety, headache, and even mild hypertension have been occasionally noted when higher doses of phenylalanine were used. Phenylalanine must be avoided by those with the rare metabolic disease phenylketonuria (PKU). Safety in young children, pregnant or nursing women, and those with liver or kidney disease has not been established. We don't know if it is safe to combine phenylalanine with standard antidepressants.

5-Hydroxytryptophan: May Be Effective, but Use Caution

A new, up-and-coming treatment for depression is 5-hydroxytryptophan (5-HTP). When the body sets about manufacturing serotonin, it first makes 5-HTP. The theory behind taking 5-HTP as a supplement is that providing the one-step-removed raw ingredient might raise serotonin levels. However, this plausible idea has not been proven.

The amino acid tryptophan used to be recommended as a treatment for depression on the same basis. It is one step back in the chain, being turned by the body into 5-HTP and then to serotonin. However, tryptophan was removed from the market several years ago when a contaminant caused a terrible and often permanent illness in many people who took the supplement. Because 5-HTP is made by a completely different manufacturing process (starting from a plant rather than a bacteria), one would not expect the same contaminant to be present. Disturbingly, however, recent reports suggest otherwise (see Safety Issues).

Like St. John's wort, 5-HTP is used mainly in Europe, where many physicians find it an effective treatment for both depression and insomnia.

What Is the Scientific Evidence for 5-HTP?

There have been several preliminary studies of 5-HTP.[24] The best of these trials was a 6-week study of 63 people given either 5-HTP (100 mg 3 times daily) or an antidepressant in the Prozac family (fluvoxamine, 50 mg 3 times daily).[25] The results showed equal benefit between the supplement and the drug. Actually, 5-HTP worked a little better, but from a mathematical perspective, the difference was not statistically significant.

5-HTP caused fewer and less severe side effects than fluvoxamine. The only real complaint was occasional mild digestive distress.

Dosage

The typical dosage of 5-HTP is 100 to 200 mg 3 times daily.

Safety Issues

5-HTP seldom causes noticeable side effects other than occasional digestive distress. However, comprehensive safety studies have not been performed, and there is one significant concern. As I mentioned earlier, the amino acid tryptophan was removed from the stores several years ago when a contaminant caused a terrible and often permanently disabling or fatal illness in many people who took the supplement. Alarmingly, on September 7, 1998, the FDA released a report stating that some commercial 5-HTP preparations had been found to contain a similar contaminant. I suggest you check with your physician for the most recent information.

Like St. John's wort, 5-HTP probably should not be combined with conventional antidepressants. Safety in young children, pregnant or nursing women, and those with severe liver or kidney disease has not been established.

Ginkgo: Improves Mental Function, but May Help Depression, Too

Ginkgo is used mainly for age-related mental decline (see the discussion of ginkgo under Alzheimer's Disease). However, during the studies on impaired mental function, researchers frequently observed improvements in mood and relief from symptoms of depression. This incidental discovery led scientists to investigate whether ginkgo might be useful as an antidepressant treatment.

One study, published in 1990, evaluated this effect in 60 people who suffered from depressive symptoms along with other signs of dementia.[26] The results showed significant improvements among participants given ginkgo extract instead of placebo.

Another study followed 40 depressed individuals over the age of 50 who had not responded successfully to antidepressant treatment.[27] Those who were given ginkgo showed an average drop of 50% in scores on the Hamilton Depression scale, whereas the placebo group showed only a 10% improvement.

In 1994 an interesting piece of research was reported that may shed light on the mechanism by which ginkgo could reduce depression.[28] This study examined levels of serotonin receptors in rats of various ages. When older rats were given ginkgo, the level of serotonin-binding sites increased. However, the same effect was not observed in younger rats. The researchers theorized that ginkgo may block an age-related loss of serotonin receptors.

Reduced receptors for serotonin may mean that the body needs more serotonin to produce a normal effect. Instead of raising the level of serotonin, like Prozac does, ginkgo may thus improve the brain's ability to respond to serotonin (at least in older people). However, this is still highly speculative. More experimentation is needed to clarify the mechanism of ginkgo's action and to better quantify its effectiveness in depression.

The proper dose of ginkgo is 40 to 80 mg of a 24% extract taken 3 times daily. As is the case with conventional antidepressants, the full benefit takes up to 6 weeks to develop.

Ginkgo appears to be very safe. Extremely high doses have been given to animals without serious consequences.[29] In all the clinical trials of ginkgo up to 1991, involving a total of almost 10,000 people, only a small number of participants reported side effects produced by ginkgo extract. There were 21 cases of gastrointestinal discomfort and even fewer cases of headaches, dizziness, and allergic skin reactions.[30]

However, because ginkgo slightly thins the blood, it should not be combined with anticoagulant drugs or even aspirin (for more information on this potential risk, see the discussion of ginkgo under Alzheimer's Disease).

Safety in young children, pregnant or nursing women, and those with severe liver or kidney disease has not been established.

Phosphatidylserine: Good for Mental
Function, May Also Help Depression

Phosphatidylserine is another treatment used mainly for mental decline in the elderly that may also offer antidepressant benefits.[31] (For more information on phosphatidylserine, see the discussion under Alzheimer's Disease.)

The proper dosage is 100 mg 3 times daily. Full results take anywhere from 4 weeks to 6 months to manifest. Although no side effects have been reported, this rather expensive supplement usually costs from $50 to $75 per month. Safety in young children, pregnant or nursing women, and those with severe liver or kidney disease has not been established.

S-Adenosylmethionine: May Be
Effective, but Very Expensive

Another European supplement treatment for depression newly arrived in the United States is S-adenosylmethionine (SAMe). SAMe is a very important biological molecule that occurs throughout the body. Its job is to hand over a chemical fragment called a methyl group to other chemicals that need it.

SAMe is especially popular in Italy, where some physicians report that it is a fast-acting antidepressant. They sometimes use SAMe alongside conventional antidepressants at the very beginning of treatment to provide immediate relief. SAMe is also used as a treatment for osteoarthritis, for which it has a fairly strong research record. Unfortunately, the sum total of evidence for SAMe as an antidepressant remains small and is flawed by the fact that most studies used an intravenous form of the supplement.

In addition to a lack of reliable evidence, SAMe is extremely expensive. The proper dosage is 400 mg 4 times daily and can cost over $200 per month. The price may come down as SAMe becomes better known.

To minimize stomach distress, most physicians recommend starting at a low dose of perhaps 200 mg twice daily and then gradually working up from there. Once you reach the full dose, stay at it for a month or so. Once you are feeling better, you can try reducing the dose again. Some physicians report that a daily dose as low as 400 mg may be effective for maintaining antidepressant benefits.

SAMe appears to be safe. However, safety in young children, pregnant or nursing women, and those with liver or kidney disease has not been established. It should not be combined with standard antidepressant treatment except under the supervision of a physician.

Vitamins and Minerals

Weak evidence suggests that the nutritional substance inositol might be helpful in depression when taken in extremely high doses (12 g daily).[32] Although this is a nutritional substance, when taken in such enormous doses safety cannot be assured.

Diets low in vitamin B_6, vitamin B_{12}, or folic acid have been associated with symptoms of depression.[33,34,35] Deficiencies of B_6 and folic acid are common, and B_{12} deficiencies occur more often with advancing age. Although there is little direct evidence that taking supplements of these vitamins will improve depression, it is important to get enough of these vitamins for your overall health anyway.

Typical daily doses are 25 to 50 mg of B_6, 400 mcg of folic acid, and 10 mcg of B_{12}. These supplements are safe when taken at these doses.

Not Recommended Treatments for Depression

The herb yohimbe and the hormone DHEA are sometimes suggested for depression, but because of potential
risks I do not suggest using them except under the supervision of a qualified health-care professional (if at all).

DIABETES

Principal Natural Treatments

Blood sugar control: Chromium, fenugreek, *Gymnema sylvestre*,
ginseng, garlic, onion, bitter melon, pterocarpus, bilberry, *Coccinia indica,* salt bush, vitamin E

Treatment of complications: Lipoic acid, evening primrose oil,
bilberry, grape seed, ginkgo, vitamin C

To correct nutritional deficiencies: Magnesium, zinc, vitamin C,
vitamin A, taurine

Diabetes has two forms. In the type that develops early in
childhood (type 1), the insulin-secreting cells of the pancreas are destroyed (probably by a viral infection), and
blood levels of insulin drop nearly to zero. However, in
the adult-onset form (type 2), insulin is often plentiful,
but the body does not respond normally to it. (This is only
an approximate description of the difference between the
two types; a full explanation is too technical for this book.)
In both forms of diabetes, blood sugar reaches toxic levels,
causing injury to many organs and tissues.

Conventional treatment for childhood-onset diabetes
includes insulin injections and careful dietary monitoring.
The adult-onset form may respond to lifestyle changes
alone, such as increasing exercise, losing weight, and improving diet. Various oral medications are also often effective for adult-onset diabetes, although insulin injections
may be necessary in some cases.

Principal Natural Treatments for Diabetes

Several alternative methods may be helpful when used under medical supervision as an addition to standard treatment. They may help stabilize, reduce, or eliminate medication requirements; reduce the symptoms of diabetic complications; or correct nutritional deficiencies associated with diabetes. (For more information, see *The Natural Pharmacist Guide to Diabetes*.) However, because diabetes is a dangerous disease with many potential complications, alternative treatment for diabetes should not be attempted as a substitute for conventional medical care.

Treatments for Improving Blood Sugar Control

The following treatments may be able to improve blood sugar control in type 1 and/or type 2 diabetes. However, keep in mind that if they work you will need to reduce your medications to avoid hypoglycemia. For this reason, medical supervision is essential.

Chromium: Helpful in Type 1 and Type 2 Diabetes

Chromium is an essential trace mineral that plays a significant role in sugar metabolism. Reasonably good evidence suggests that chromium supplementation may help bring blood sugar levels under control in both type 1 and type 2 diabetes.

A 4-month study reported in 1997 followed 180 Chinese men and women with type 2 diabetes, comparing the effects of 1,000 mcg chromium, 200 mcg chromium, and a placebo.[1] The results showed that HbA1c values (a measure of long-term blood sugar control) improved significantly after 2 months in the group receiving 1,000 mcg, and in both chromium groups after 4 months. Fasting glucose was also lower in the group taking the higher dose of chromium.

Another controlled study in 1993 of 243 people with either type 1 or type 2 diabetes found that chromium supplementation at 200 mcg daily decreased insulin, or oral medication, requirements in 57% of adult-onset and 34% of childhood-onset cases.[2] More women than men responded favorably, and placebo was ineffective. While not all studies have produced positive results,[3] the bulk of the evidence suggests that chromium is indeed effective.

The optimum dosage of chromium is not known. The usual recommended dosage is 400 to 600 mcg daily (as chromium picolinate). However, one of the recent studies just described used a higher dose. Since there have been a few worrisome case reports of toxic effects when chromium has been taken at daily doses of 1,200 mcg or higher[4,5] you should consult with your physician on what might be the appropriate dosage for you.

Fenugreek: Appears to Be Helpful

The food spice fenugreek may also help control blood sugar. For millennia, fenugreek has been used both as a medicine and as a spice in Egypt, India, and the Middle East. Numerous animal studies and small-scale trials in humans involving a total of about 100 people have found that fenugreek can reduce blood sugar and serum cholesterol levels in people with diabetes.[6,7,8] It seems to be helpful in both type 1 and type 2 diabetes.

Dosage Because the seeds of fenugreek are somewhat bitter, fenugreek is best taken in capsule form. The typical dosage is 5 to 30 g 3 times a day with meals, taken indefinitely.

Safety Issues As a commonly eaten food, fenugreek is generally regarded as safe. The only common side effect is mild gastrointestinal distress when it is taken in high doses.

Extracts made from fenugreek have been shown to cause uterine contractions in guinea pigs.[9] For this reason, pregnant women should not take fenugreek in doses higher than is commonly used as a spice, perhaps 5 g daily. Safety in young children, nursing women, or those with severe liver or kidney disease has also not been established.

Gymnema sylvestre: Early Evidence Suggests It Is Effective

A few preliminary studies suggest that the Ayurvedic (Indian) herb *Gymnema sylvestre* may help improve blood sugar control.[10,11,12] In practice, many clinicians report that gymnema is more powerful than the other treatments described in this section.

The recommended dose of gymnema ranges from 400 mg to 2 g daily. Because no formal safety studies have been conducted, gymnema should not be taken by young children, pregnant or nursing women, or those with severe kidney or liver disease.

Ginseng: Promising New Evidence

A double-blind study evaluated the effects of ginseng in 36 people newly diagnosed with adult-onset diabetes over an 8-week period.[13] The results showed a reduction in glucose levels, improved glycosylated hemoglobin (a measure of long-term blood sugar control), and improved physical capacity. Although ginseng is generally believed to be safe, safety in young children, pregnant or nursing women, and those with severe kidney or liver disease has not been established. (See Colds and Flus for a more detailed discussion of the potential safety issues associated with ginseng.)

Other Treatments That May Help Control Blood Sugar

Preliminary evidence suggests that the herbs garlic, onion, bitter melon, pterocarpus, bilberry, *Coccinia indica*, and salt bush may help some people with diabetes improve blood sugar control.[14–26] (For more information, see *The Natural Pharmacist Guide to Diabetes.*)

Preliminary studies indicate that vitamin E may also slightly improve blood sugar control in type 2 diabetes.[27,28] (For a discussion of the safety and proper dosage of vitamin E, see Atherosclerosis.)

Treating Complications of Diabetes

Several supplements may help prevent or treat some of the common complications of diabetes.

Because atherosclerosis is one of the worst problems with diabetes, all the suggestions discussed under Atherosclerosis may be useful.

Other herbs and supplements may be helpful for diabetic neuropathy, diabetic retinopathy, and diabetic cataracts (see also the discussion under Cataracts).

Lipoic Acid: Standard German Treatment for Diabetic Neuropathy

Lipoic acid has been widely used in Germany for over 20 years to treat diabetic peripheral neuropathy, a painful nerve condition that often develops after many years of diabetes. This naturally occurring antioxidant may also help prevent and treat cardiac autonomic neuropathy (injury to the nerves controlling the heart) and diabetic cataracts.

Lipoic acid is a vitamin-like substance that plays a role in the body's utilization of energy. Because lipoic acid can be synthesized from other substances, it is not considered an essential nutrient. However, in people with diabetes, levels of lipoic acid are reduced.[29] It is not clear whether lipoic acid supplements correct a deficiency or whether they work in some other way.

What Is the Scientific Evidence for Lipoic Acid? Several double-blind studies support the use of lipoic acid for diabetic neuropathy.[30,31]

In the ALADIN (Alpha-Lipoic Acid in Diabetic Neuropathy) study, 328 people were randomized into four groups and given either a placebo or 100, 600, or 1,200 mg intravenous lipoic acid daily. Over a course of 3 weeks, the participants were assessed for improvements in sensations such as pain and numbness. The results showed greatest improvement in the 600 mg group, with 82.5% showing adequate response compared to only 57.6% in the placebo group. (As always, the power of placebo is remarkable!) Unfortunately, because in this study the lipoic acid was injected, it is not clear whether the results carry over to oral lipoic acid.

Warning: Do not inject lipoic acid products intended for oral use.

Another study used oral lipoic acid. In this 3-month trial, 80 people with diabetes were divided into four groups and treated with oral lipoic acid (660 mg daily), selenium (100 mcg daily), vitamin E (1,200 IU daily), or placebo.[32] Again, lipoic acid significantly improved symptoms compared to the placebo.

However, in this study, vitamin E and selenium worked just as well as lipoic acid. This finding gives rise to a suspicion that it may be possible to use cheaper antioxidants instead of lipoic acid. (For more information on the safe use of vitamin E and selenium, see *The Natural Pharmacist: Your Complete Guide to Vitamins and Supplements.*)

The DEKAN (Deutsche Kardiale Autonome Neuropathie) study followed 73 people with diabetes, who had symptoms of cardiac autonomic neuropathy, for 4 months.[33] Treatment with 800 mg of oral lipoic acid daily showed significant improvement compared to placebo and no important side effects.

Dosage The typical dosage of lipoic acid for diabetic peripheral neuropathy is 300 to 600 mg daily, divided into

2 or 3 doses. For cardiac autonomic neuropathy, a higher dosage of 800 mg daily has been used in studies.

Because lipoic acid occasionally improves the body's response to insulin, it may be necessary to start with lower doses and gradually increase while monitoring blood sugar levels under a physician's supervision.

Safety Issues Over the 30 years during which lipoic acid has been used for diabetic peripheral neuropathy in Germany, no serious adverse reactions have been reported. Side effects are rare and generally limited to mild gastrointestinal distress. However, safety in young children, pregnant or nursing women, and those with severe kidney or liver disease has not been established.

Evening Primrose Oil: Probably Helpful, but Slow-Acting

Evening primrose is a native American wildflower, named for the late-afternoon opening of its delicate flowers. Perhaps it should be described as a food supplement rather than an herb, for evening primrose oil (EPO) has been popularized mainly as a source of gamma-linolenic acid (GLA), an essential fatty acid also found in black currant and borage oil.

Although many other kinds of fat are unhealthy, essential fatty acids (EFAs) are as necessary as vitamins. The two main kinds of EFAs are called omega-3 and omega-6 fatty acids. The GLA in EPO is an omega-6 fatty acid. A growing body of scientific evidence suggests that supplementation with GLA may help relieve symptoms of diabetic neuropathy.

What Is the Scientific Evidence for EPO? Many studies in animals have shown that EPO can protect nerves from diabetes-induced injury.[34,35] Good results were also seen in a double-blind study that followed 111 people with diabetes from seven medical centers for a period of 1 year.[36] The results showed an improvement in subjective symptoms such as pain and numbness as well as objective signs of nerve injury. Individuals with good blood sugar control improved the most. Earlier double-blind studies also reported positive results.[37]

Dosage A typical dosage of EPO for diabetic neuropathy is 4 to 6 g daily. It should be taken with food. Keep in mind that full results may take over 6 months to develop.

Safety Issues Animal studies suggest that EPO is nontoxic and noncarcinogenic.[38] Over 4,000 people have taken GLA or EPO in scientific studies, and no significant adverse effects have ever been noted.

Somewhat less than 2% of people who take EPO complain of mild headaches, gastrointestinal distress, or both, especially at higher doses.[39,40]

Early case reports suggested the possibility that GLA might worsen temporal lobe epilepsy or bipolar disorder, but this has not been confirmed.[41,42]

Maximum safe dosages in young children, pregnant or nursing women, and those with severe kidney or liver disease have not been established.

Other Treatments to Help Treat Complications of Diabetes
Weak evidence suggests that the herb bilberry (120 to 240 mg twice daily of an extract standardized to contain 25% anthocyanosides) may help prevent eye damage caused by diabetes, especially when it is taken with vitamin E.[43,44] (For a more complete discussion of bilberry use and safety issues, see the discussion under Night Vision.)

Grape seed extract and ginkgo are said to provide similar benefits, although the evidence for these is weaker than that of bilberry. (See Varicose Veins and Alzheimer's Disease for more complete discussions of grape seed PCOs and ginkgo, respectively.)

Vitamin C is believed to help prevent cataracts in general.[45,46] It is not known for sure whether vitamin C produces the same benefit in people with diabetes. However, it has been suggested that vitamin C may actually be especially useful because of its relationship to sorbitol, a sugar-like substance that tends to accumulate in the cells of people with diabetes. Sorbitol is believed to play a role in the development of diabetic cataracts, and vitamin C appears to help reduce sorbitol buildup.[47] However, the evidence that vitamin C provides significant benefits through this route is at present indirect and far from conclusive. A daily dose of 500 mg should be safe and sufficient.

Treating Nutritional Deficiencies in Diabetes

Both diabetes and the medications used to treat it can cause people to fall short of various nutrients. Making up for these deficiencies (either through diet or the use of supplements) may not help your diabetes, but it should make you a healthier person overall.

Magnesium appears to be the most common mineral deficiency in type 1 diabetes.[48,49] People with either type 1 or type 2 diabetes may also be deficient in the mineral zinc.[50,51,52] Vitamin C levels have been found to be low in many diabetics on insulin, even though they were consuming seemingly adequate amounts in their diets.[53,54,55] Vitamin A has been found to be depleted in the bloodstream of diabetics as compared to nondiabetics,[56] partly because of difficulties in getting vitamin A out of the liver, where it is stored.[57,58] Finally, some people with type 1 diabetes appear to be deficient in the amino acid taurine.[59]

Dosage and Safety Issues

So that you do not take unnecessary supplements, you may want to undergo testing to determine whether you are actually deficient in any of these nutrients. However, such testing is expensive. Because these are safe supplements, you may want to take them simply as insurance.

Typical dosages for nutritional correction are as follows: magnesium, 350 mg daily; zinc 15 to 30 mg daily (combined with 1 to 3 mg daily of copper); vitamin C, 500 mg daily; and taurine, 1.5 g daily. Supplementation with vitamin A is generally recommended at a dose of about 5,000 IU daily; however, women who are or who may become pregnant should take no more than 2,500 IU. A general multivitamin and mineral may not be a bad idea, either, for there may be many other marginal deficiencies in diabetes. However, if you suffer from diabetic kidney disease, you should not take any supplements except on the advice of a physician.

People with diabetes should not take high doses of niacin, as it can worsen blood sugar control.

DYSMENORRHEA
(Painful Menstruation)

Principal Natural Treatments
Fish oil
Other Natural Treatments
Magnesium, cramp bark, turmeric, white willow, bromelain

We do not know why menstruation is uncomfortable at all, or why it is much more painful for some women than for others and varies so much from month to month.

Occasionally, severe menstrual pain indicates the presence of endometriosis (a condition in which uterine tissue is growing in places other than the uterus) or uterine fibroids (benign tumors in the uterus), but in most cases no such identifiable abnormality can be found. Natural substances known as prostaglandins seem to play a central role in menstrual pain, but the details of the many interactions are scarcely understood, and the available treatments are not specific in their action.

Anti-inflammatory drugs such as ibuprofen usually relieve menstrual pain substantially. However, their blood-thinning effects can increase menstrual flow. Oral contraceptive treatment can also help over the long term, although its success is not guaranteed.

Principal Natural Treatments for Dysmenorrhea

The best evidence we have for any treatment for dysmenorrhea is in regards to fish oil.

Fish Oil: Appears to Relieve Cramps

Fish oil supplements, a good source of omega-3 fatty acids, appear to be quite helpful for the treatment of painful menstruation.

In a 2-month study of 42 adolescents aged 15 to 18, fish oil significantly reduced menstrual pain.[1] Half received 6 g daily of fish oil, providing 1,080 mg of eicosapentaenoic acid (EPA) and 720 mg of docosahexaenoic acid (DHA) daily for 2 months. This was followed by a placebo for 2 months. The other half received the same treatments in the reverse order. The girls in the study reported improvements in their symptoms while they were taking fish oil, but not when they were taking placebo. It is believed that the omega-3 fatty acids in fish oil may help relieve dysmenorrhea by affecting the metabolism of prostaglandins and other factors involved in pain and inflammation.[2]

There are many different types of fish oil products available. A typical daily dose should supply about 1,000 to 2,000 mg of EPA and 500 to 750 mg of DHA. Cod liver oil is probably not the best choice due to the potential for excessive intake of vitamin A and D. Flaxseed oil has been proposed as a less smelly alternative to fish oil, but it has not been proven effective.

Side effects, other than fishy burps, are rare.

Other Natural Treatments for Dysmenorrhea

The following natural treatments are widely recommended for painful menstruation, but none have been scientifically proven effective at this time.

Magnesium

Preliminary studies suggest that magnesium supplementation may be helpful for dysmenorrhea.[3,4] A typical dosage is 350 to 500 mg daily throughout the cycle, or 500 to 1,000 mg for 3 to 5 days prior to the onset of cramps. Magnesium is described in more detail in the discussion under PMS.

Other Herbs

The herb cramp bark has traditionally been used to relieve menstrual pain. Unfortunately, it has not received any significant scientific attention.

Herbs with possible anti-inflammatory properties may be helpful as well, including turmeric, white willow, and bromelain.

ECZEMA

Principal Natural Treatments

Evening primrose oil

Other Natural Treatments

Topical herbal creams, burdock, red clover, zinc

Eczema is an allergic reaction shown in the skin. It consists mainly of itchy, inflamed patches on the face, elbows, knees, and wrists. Eczema is most commonly found in infants and young children, and many children with eczema also develop hay fever and asthma.

Medical treatment for eczema consists mainly of topical steroid creams.

Principal Natural Treatments for Eczema

Evening primrose oil is widely used in Europe for eczema, although the evidence that it really works is mixed.

Evening Primrose Oil:
Standard Treatment for Eczema in Europe

A review of all studies reported up to 1989 found that EPO frequently reduced the symptoms of eczema after several months of use, with the greatest improvement noticeable in the level of itching.[1] However, this review has been criticized because it used unpublished studies as well as studies of poor design.[2] A recent properly designed double-blind study that followed 58 children with eczema for 16 weeks found no difference between the treated and placebo groups.[3] Another double-blind trial followed 39 people with hand dermatitis (inflammation) for 24 weeks. EPO at a dosage of 6 g daily produced no significant improvement as compared to the placebo.[4]

A 1985 double-blind study of 123 individuals with moderately severe eczema also found no benefits, but this study appears to have mixed up the treatment and placebo groups![5,6,7]

One recent double-blind trial did find a therapeutic benefit with EPO.[8] Putting all this information together, it appears likely that evening primrose oil may be mildly effective for eczema.

The typical dosage of EPO is 2 to 4 g daily, taken with food. Full results are said to take over 6 months to develop. Combinations of fish oil and EPO may be more effective. EPO is believed to be quite safe.

Other Natural Treatments for Eczema

The following natural treatments are widely recommended for eczema, but they have not been scientifically proven effective at this time.

Topical Herbal Creams

Topical creams made from chamomile, licorice, or calendula, alone or in combination, are also widely used in Europe to treat eczema.

Burdock and Red Clover

The herbs burdock and red clover are traditionally drunk as tea to treat eczema. The proper dosage of these herbs varies according to the preparation, so follow the label instructions.

Burdock is a common food in Japan (it is often found in sukiyaki) and as such is believed to be safe.

The safety of red clover is less clear because it contains many blood-thinning and estrogen-like substances. It may not be appropriate for long-term use, especially in girls and adolescents; and it should not be taken by pregnant or nursing women and those on anticoagulant drugs, such as Coumadin (warfarin), Trental (pentoxifylline), or even aspirin.

Zinc

Zinc supplementation is said to be effective for eczema in some children. The usual dosage is 10 mg of zinc picolinate daily in children under 10, balanced with 1 mg of copper. For older individuals, the dosage is 15 to 30 mg taken daily, balanced with 1 to 3 mg of copper daily. Too much zinc can be toxic, so dosages should not exceed 30 mg daily.

GALLSTONES

Principal Natural Treatments

There are no well-established natural treatments for gallstones.

Other Natural Treatments

Peppermint, milk thistle, artichoke leaf, boldo, fumitory, greater celandine, turmeric, dandelion

The job of the gallbladder is to store the bile produced by the liver and to release it on an as-needed basis for digestive purposes. However, it isn't easy to keep this complex mixture of chemicals in liquid form. The various elements of bile have a natural tendency to form sludge, lumps, and hard deposits called gallstones. The body uses several biochemical methods to prevent such condensation from occurring, but this natural chemistry does not always succeed. More than 20% of women and 8% of men develop gallstones at some time in their lives.

You could have gallstones in your body for many years without experiencing any problems. According to current medical guidelines, no treatment is necessary unless pain or other problems begin to develop. However, when a gallstone plugs the duct that leads out of the gallbladder, the organ becomes inflamed and often infected, creating a condition known as cholecystitis.

Generally, gallbladder pain begins with occasional minor attacks that subside rapidly. Perhaps the stones are blocking the duct temporarily and then moving out of the way. However, when full obstruction occurs, the pain often becomes severe and recurrent.

The most reliable symptom of cholecystitis is intense pain beneath the right lower rib cage, often occurring from midnight to 3 A.M. Typically, pain radiates to the right shoulder and is accompanied by a loss of appetite and sometimes nausea. Frequently, fatty meals seem to bring on the pain with particular force.

Techniques for removing the gallbladder have become quite sophisticated. Today, the gallbladder can be removed quickly and usually without complications, bringing full relief of symptoms.

Living without a gallbladder does not seem to bring any long-term consequences. However, many people are opposed on general principle to removing an organ that nature has placed there. The medication Actigall may be able to dissolve gallstones when it is taken for many months.

Natural Treatments for Gallstones

The only time it is appropriate to use alternative treatments for gallstones is before acute cholecystitis develops. Once the gallbladder has become completely blocked, there is a real danger of imminent rupture. Another risk is that a stone may escape the gallbladder and obstruct the common bile duct. When this happens, the liver cannot unload the bile it produces, putting it at risk of permanent injury and creating a true surgical emergency.

However, during the period in which pain is only occasional or intermittent, the risks incurred by postponing surgery are slight. During the same interval when the medication Actigall might be tried, some of the agents described here could be considered as possibilities. Unfortunately, none are well established as effective. Medical supervision is definitely essential.

Peppermint

Preliminary clinical trials suggest that formulas containing peppermint and related terpenes (fragrant substances found in plants) can dissolve gallstones.[1] The proper dosage is not clear, but a typical recommendation is 1 or 2 capsules containing 0.2 ml of peppermint oil 3 times daily. The label should say "enteric coated," meaning that it remains intact until it has passed the stomach. Excessive doses of peppermint oil can cause severe gastrointestinal distress and other symptoms, so do not take more than this amount.

Milk Thistle

Milk thistle, standardized to its silymarin content, has been shown to improve the liquidity of bile,[2] although its actual effects on gallstones in real life is unknown. The proper dosage should provide about 140 to 210 mg of silymarin to be taken 3 times daily. (For more information on milk thistle use and safety issues, see the discussion under Hepatitis.)

Other European Herbs

Other herbs that are widely prescribed in Germany for gallbladder pain include artichoke leaf, boldo, fumitory, greater celandine, turmeric, and dandelion.[3]

Consult a qualified physician before using these substances, as they can cause increased pain and may present other risks.

GOUT

Principal Natural Treatments

There are no well-established natural treatments for gout.

Other Natural Treatments

Folic acid, devil's claw, fish oil, flaxseed oil, vitamin E, selenium, quercetin, bromelain, aspartic acid, cherry juice, celery juice

Gout is an inflammatory condition that is caused by the deposit of uric acid crystals in joints (most famously the big toe) as well as other tissues. Typically, attacks of fierce pain, redness, swelling, and heat punctuate pain-free intervals.

Medical treatment consists of anti-inflammatory drugs for acute attacks and of uric acid–lowering drugs for prevention.

Natural Treatments for Gout

The following herbs and supplements are widely recommended for gout, but they have not yet been scientifically proven effective.

Folic Acid

Folic acid has been recommended as a preventive treatment for gout for at least 20 years. Some clinicians report that it can be highly effective. However, what little scientific evidence we have on the method is contradictory.[1,2,3] It has been suggested that a contaminant found in folic acid, pterin-6-aldehyde, may actually be responsible for the positive effects observed by some clinicians.

A typical dosage of folic acid for gout is 10 mg daily. However, because folic acid can mask vitamin B_{12} deficiency, it is important to consult with a qualified health-care practitioner before using this method. High doses of folic acid can also cause digestive distress and may worsen seizures in epileptics. The safety of high doses of folic acid in young children, pregnant or nursing women, and those with severe kidney or liver disease has not been established.

Devil's Claw

The herb devil's claw is sometimes recommended as a pain-relieving treatment for gout based on evidence for its effectiveness in various forms of arthritis.[4] A typical dosage is 750 mg 3 times daily of a preparation standardized to contain 3% iridoid glycosides.

Devil's claw appears to be quite safe, and there is no evidence of toxicity at dosages many times higher than recommended. However, safety in pregnant or nursing women and those with severe liver or kidney disease has not been established. It is not recommended for use by those with ulcers, as it can sometimes cause stomach irritation.

It is not known whether devil's claw interacts with any drugs.

Other Supplements

On the basis of interesting reasoning but no concrete evidence of effectiveness, fish oil, flaxseed oil, vitamin E, selenium, quercetin, bromelain, and aspartic acid have also been recommended for both prevention and treatment of gout.[5]

Folk Remedies

A traditional remedy for gout (with negligible scientific evidence) calls for ½ to 1 pound of cherries a day.[6] You can also buy tablets containing concentrated cherry juice.

Celery juice is another folk remedy for gout that is said to be widely used in Australia.

HEMORRHOIDS

Principal Natural Treatments

Hydroxyethylrutosides

Other Natural Treatments

Aortic glycosaminoglycans, collinsonia, horse chestnut, grape seed PCOs, gotu kola, butcher's broom, bilberry

Hemorrhoids are swollen, inflamed veins in the rectum that can ache and bleed. They are very common and are usually caused by constipation, a low-fiber diet, a sedentary lifestyle, or pregnancy.

The most important interventions for hemorrhoids aim at reversing their causes. Adopting a high-fiber diet, sitting down less, getting plenty of exercise, and maintaining regular bowel habits can make a significant difference.

Medical treatment consists mainly of stool softeners and moist heat. In more severe cases, surgical procedures may be used.

Principal Natural Treatments for Hemorrhoids

Besides the treatments described in this section, the natural treatments used for varicose veins are also often recommended for hemorrhoids because hemorrhoids are actually a special kind of varicose vein. These include horse chestnut, grape seed PCOs, gotu kola, butcher's broom, and bilberry.

Bioflavonoids

Bioflavonoids are colorful substances that occur widely in the plant kingdom. A certain category of bioflavonoid, called hydroxyethylrutosides (HERs), is extensively used in Europe to relieve hemorrhoid pain. Preliminary double-blind studies suggest that these safe substances can be beneficial in cases of hemorrhoids, including those that occur during pregnancy.[1,2,3]

These naturally occurring substances are considered very safe, as shown by the fact that researchers felt comfortable giving them to pregnant women. Typical dosages are 500 to 1,000 mg 2 or 3 times daily.

Although it is not known precisely how flavonoids work, it has been suggested that they stabilize the walls of blood vessels, making them less susceptible to injury.

Other Natural Treatments for Hemorrhoids

The following natural treatments are widely recommended for hemorrhoids, but they have not been scientifically proven effective at this time.

Aortic Glycosaminoglycans

Preliminary evidence suggests that an extract made from the inner lining of cow aortas called aortic glycosaminoglycans (GAGs) can improve the symptoms of hemorrhoids.[4,5] The recommended dosage is 50 mg twice daily.

Collinsonia

Collinsonia root (also known as stone root) is a traditional remedy for hemorrhoids. The proper dosage varies according to the preparation and is usually listed on the label. Safety studies have not been performed.

HEPATITIS
(Viral)

Principal Natural Treatments
Milk thistle
Other Natural Treatments
Licorice, Chinese and Japanese herb combinations, vitamin C, liver extracts, thymus extracts, *Phyllanthus amarus*

Hepatitis is an infection of the liver caused by one of several viruses, the most common of which are named hepatitis A, B, and C. Hepatitis A is spread mainly through contaminated food and water, whereas hepatitis B is transmitted by sexual contact and use of contaminated needles. The route of transmission of hepatitis C is not completely clear but is believed to be similar to that of hepatitis B.

When you first develop hepatitis, it is called acute hepatitis. Hepatitis can also become a long-term disease known as chronic hepatitis. All forms of hepatitis cause jaundice, liver tenderness, and severe fatigue. Hepatitis A is the mildest form and seldom causes symptoms continuing longer than a couple of months. Hepatitis B and C produce more severe symptoms, last two or three times longer, and can go on to become chronic.

Chronic hepatitis consists of persistent liver infection and inflammation that lingers long after the primary symptoms of the disease have disappeared. It can produce subtle symptoms of liver tenderness and continued fatigue and over time can gradually destroy the liver. Chronic hepatitis also appears to increase the risk of liver cancer.

The best treatment for hepatitis is prevention. You can avoid hepatitis A by practicing good hygiene and using the conventional treatment, known as immune globulins, while traveling in areas where the disease is common. Hepatitis B can be prevented by immunization and the same precautions taken against AIDS. AIDS precautions almost certainly decrease the transmission of hepatitis C as well.

Conventional medicine has little in the way of treatment for the initial hepatitis infection once it has started. Treatment for chronic hepatitis is developing but is still quite imperfect. The most effective methods involve varieties of interferon.

Principal Natural Treatments for Hepatitis

In Europe, the herb milk thistle is commonly used along with other treatments for hepatitis. Keep in mind, though, that this is a very serious disease. Medical supervision is essential.

Milk Thistle: May Be Helpful for Chronic Hepatitis

The herb milk thistle may be useful as a supportive treatment for chronic hepatitis. Native to Europe and the United States, milk thistle has a long history of use as both a food and a medicine. At the turn of the twentieth century, English gardeners grew milk thistle to use its leaves like lettuce, the stalks like asparagus, the roasted seeds like coffee, and the roots (soaked overnight) like oyster plant. The seeds, fruit, and leaves of milk thistle are also used for medicinal purposes.

German researchers in the 1960s were sufficiently impressed with the history and clinical effectiveness of milk thistle to begin examining it for active constituents. The most important ingredient appears to be silymarin (actually a set of four related substances), which appears to possess a wide variety of liver-protective benefits. It is one of the few herbs that has no real equivalent among standard medications.

In 1986, Germany's Commission E approved an oral extract of milk thistle standardized to 70% silymarin content as a treatment for "toxic liver damage; also the supportive treatment of chronic inflammatory liver diseases and hepatic cirrhosis." The herb is widely used in chronic viral hepatitis as well as alcoholic fatty liver, liver cirrhosis, alcoholic hepatitis, chemical-induced liver toxicity, and abnormal liver enzymes of unknown cause. In addition, milk thistle is often added as a protective agent when drugs that are known to be toxic to the liver are used. An intravenous preparation made from milk thistle is used as an antidote for poisoning by the deathcap mushroom, *Amanita phalloides.*

For more information on the general liver-protective effects of milk thistle, see *The Natural Pharmacist: Your Complete Guide to Herbs.* I will concentrate here on the evidence for its use in chronic hepatitis.

What Is the Scientific Evidence for Milk Thistle?

Preliminary double-blind studies of people with chronic hepatitis have shown significant improvement in symptoms such as fatigue, reduced appetite, and abdominal discomfort.[1,2,3] Laboratory signs of liver injury also showed improvement in these trials. However, larger research trials need to be performed before milk thistle can be called a proven treatment for chronic hepatitis. Milk thistle is probably not helpful during the initial acute hepatitis infection.[4]

As for most herbs, the mechanism of action of milk thistle remains in doubt. In mushroom poisoning and other liver-toxic exposure, silymarin is believed to get in the way of toxins trying to bind to liver cell membrane receptors by binding to the receptors itself.[5] This is called *competitive inhibition.* Incidentally, glutathione, a compound that our body normally produces to protect the liver and kidney from reactive chemicals, works in a similar fashion. Many other suggestions of how milk thistle may function have been made, but which one is correct remains unclear.[6–10]

Dosage

The standard dosage of milk thistle is 200 mg 2 or 3 times daily of an extract standardized to contain 70% silymarin.

Some evidence supports the idea that silymarin bound to phosphatidylcholine is better absorbed.[11,12] This form should be taken at a dosage of 100 to 200 mg twice daily.

Safety Issues

Milk thistle is believed to possess very little toxicity. Animal studies have not shown any negative effects even when high doses were administered over a long period of time.[13]

A study of 2,637 participants reported in 1992 showed a low incidence of side effects, limited mainly to mild gastrointestinal disturbance.[14]

On the basis of its extensive use as a food, milk thistle is believed to be safe in pregnancy and lactation (milk production), and researchers have enrolled pregnant women in studies.[15] However, safety in young children, pregnant or nursing women, and individuals with severe renal disease has not been formally established. No drug interactions are known.

One report has noted that silibinin (a constituent of silymarin) can inhibit a bacterial enzyme called beta-glucuronidase, which plays a role in the activity of certain drugs, such as oral contraceptives.[16] This could interfere with their action.

Other Natural Treatments for Hepatitis

The following natural treatments are widely recommended for hepatitis, but they have not been scientifically proven effective at this time.

Licorice

In Japan, an injectable combination of licorice (the herb, not the candy) and certain amino acids is used for chronic hepatitis.[17] However, it is not clear whether oral licorice is equally useful, and the high dosages used for treatment of chronic hepatitis may cause an elevation of blood pressure.

Warning: Do not inject preparations of licorice designed for oral use.

Herb Combinations

Chinese and Japanese herbal medicine typically use combinations of herbs rather than just one. A multicenter, randomized, controlled clinical study looked at the effectiveness of a combination containing the herb *Radix bupleuri* in chronic hepatitis and found good results.[18] However, this combination has not been formally tested to verify its safety.

Other Herbs and Supplements

Other common natural medicine recommendations for hepatitis include high doses of vitamin C, liver extracts, thymus extracts, and the herb *Phyllanthus amarus*. However, the scientific evidence that these approaches really work is contradictory at best.

HERPES
(Genital Herpes and Cold Sores)

Principal Natural Treatments
Melissa officinalis, L-lysine
Other Natural Treatments
Vitamin C

The common virus known as herpes can cause painful blister-like lesions around the mouth and in the genitalia. Slightly different strains of herpes predominate in each of these two locations, but the infections are essentially identical. In both areas, the herpes virus has the devious habit of hiding out deep in the DNA of nerve ganglia, where it remains inactive for months or years. From time to time the virus reactivates, travels down the nerve, and starts an eruption. Common triggers include stress, dental procedures, infections, and trauma. Flare-ups usually become less severe over time.

Conventional medical treatment consists of antiviral drugs, such as Zovirax. Such medications can shorten the length and intensity of a herpes outbreak or, when taken consistently at lower dosages, reduce the frequency of flare-ups. However, they are not dramatically effective.

Principal Natural Treatments for Herpes

The herb *Melissa officinalis* and the amino acid L-lysine appear to be effective treatments for herpes.

Melissa officinalis *(Lemon Balm)*

More commonly known in the United States as lemon balm, *Melissa officinalis* is widely sold in Europe as a topical cream for the treatment of genital and oral herpes. This herb is a native of southern Europe and is widely planted in gardens for the purpose of attracting bees. Its leaves give off a delicate lemon odor when bruised.

Melissa cream appears to be helpful in the treatment of genital and oral herpes. It can be applied only at the first sign of blisters or on a regular basis for the prevention of flare-ups. However, there is no evidence that melissa will stop you from infecting another person.

What Is the Scientific Evidence for Melissa?

A double-blind placebo-controlled trial involving 116 people found that treatment with melissa cream helped the herpes blisters heal more rapidly.[1] The total number of participants who were completely recovered on the fifth day was 24 of 58 in the melissa group but only 15 of 58 in the placebo group, a statistically significant difference.

The regular use of melissa cream may also decrease the frequency of recurrences.[2]

The most commonly used European melissa product is manufactured using a method that tests the herb's activity against the herpes virus. Here's how it's designed: Human or animal cells are grown in a petri dish and then infected with herpes virus. Left alone, the virus would gradually spread throughout the dish, killing all the cells. However, in this test, standard paper disks containing melissa extract are inserted into the petri dish. The commercial extract is standardized so that a dose of 200 mcg per disk forms a 20 to 30 mm (millimeter) zone of protection from the virus.[3]

We don't really know how melissa works. The leading theory is that the herb makes it more difficult for the herpes virus to attach to cells.

Dosage

For treatment of an active flare-up of herpes, the proper dosage is four thick daily applications of a standard melissa 70:1 extract cream. This can be reduced to twice daily for preventive purposes.

Pregnant women should not regard melissa as effective prevention against transmission to the newborn. It also will not prevent spread of the disease in sexually active individuals.

Safety Issues

Topical melissa is not associated with any significant side effects, although allergic reactions are always possible. Safety in young children, pregnant or nursing women, and those with severe liver or kidney disease has not been established.

L-Lysine

Another famous treatment for herpes involves the amino acid L-lysine. Although study results have been somewhat contradictory, overall the evidence from several double-blind studies suggests that adequate doses of L-lysine can make herpes flare-ups milder and less frequent.[4] Lysine probably works best when it is combined with dietary changes that restrict levels of another amino acid, arginine. (To do this, cut down on gelatin, chocolate, peanuts, almonds and other nuts, seeds, and to a lesser extent wheat.)

A double-blind placebo-controlled trial tested the efficacy of L-lysine in preventing recurring herpes simplex.[5] Twenty-seven individuals were given 1,000 mg of L-lysine 3 times a day for 6 months, while 25 subjects received placebo. Those treated with L-lysine experienced, on average, 2.4 fewer herpes flare-ups than the placebo group, a significant result. The L-lysine group also experienced significantly less severe flare-ups and shorter healing time.

Another placebo-controlled double-blind study on 41 subjects found that 1,250 mg of L-lysine per day also worked, but 624 mg did not.[6] One study found no benefit, but it was very small.[7]

Foods high in L-lysine include vegetables, beans, fish, turkey, and chicken. When taken as a supplement, a typical daily dose is 1,000 mg. L-lysine in supplement form has not been associated with any significant side effects. However, high doses of L-lysine in animals have caused gallstones and elevated cholesterol levels.[8,9]

Other Natural Treatments for Herpes

The following natural treatments are widely recommended for herpes, but they have not been scientifically proven effective at this time.

Vitamin C

One study suggests that topical treatment with a vitamin C solution may speed healing of herpes outbreaks.[10]

Oral vitamin C may also be useful, especially when combined with bioflavonoids.[11] A typical dose is 200 mg of vitamin C combined with 200 mg of mixed bioflavonoids, taken 5 times daily at the very first signs of an impending outbreak. Short-term use of these substances has not been associated with any significant risks.

HYPERTENSION
(High Blood Pressure)

Principal Natural Treatments
Garlic, coenzyme Q_{10}

Other Natural Treatments
Fish oil, calcium, magnesium, potassium, hawthorn, vitamin C

Most people can't tell when their blood pressure is high, which is why hypertension is called the "silent killer." In this case, what you don't know can hurt you. Elevated blood pressure can lead to a greatly increased risk of heart attack, stroke, and many other serious illnesses. Along with high cholesterol and smoking, hypertension is one of the most important causes of atherosclerosis (hardening of the arteries). In turn, atherosclerosis causes heart attacks, strokes, and other diseases of impaired circulation.

The mechanism by which high blood pressure produces atherosclerosis is similar to a hose fitted with a high-pressure nozzle. All such nozzles come with a warning label that states, "Make sure to discharge pressure in hose after using." Unfortunately, many people (such as myself) frequently fail to pay attention to the warning and leave the hose puffed up with full pressure overnight.

This rather common practice does not produce any immediate consequences. The hose doesn't develop leaks at the seams or burst outright on the first occasion you leave it untended. However, a garden hose that is frequently left under pressure will begin to age more rapidly than it would otherwise. Its lining will begin to crack, its flexibility will diminish, and within a season or two the hose will be sprouting leaks in all directions.

When blood vessels are exposed to constantly high pressure, a similar process is set in motion. Blood pressures as elevated as 220/170 (systolic pressure/diastolic pressure), quite common during activities such as weightlifting, do no harm. Only when excessive pressure is sustained day and night do blood vessel linings begin to be injured and undergo those unhealthy changes known as hardening of the arteries, or atherosclerosis (see Atherosclerosis for more information).

Thus, although it is important to lower blood pressure with all deliberate speed, only rarely does it need to be lowered instantly. In most situations, you have plenty of time to work on bringing down your blood pressure. However, that doesn't mean that you should ignore it. Over time, high blood pressure can damage nearly every organ in the body.

The best way to determine your blood pressure is to take several readings at different times of the day and on different days of the week. Blood pressure readings will vary quite a bit from moment to moment; what matters most is the average blood pressure. Thus, if many low readings balance out a few high readings, the net result may be satisfactory.

However, it is essential not to ignore a high value by saying, "I was just stressed then." Stress is part of life, and if it raises your blood pressure once, it will do so again. To come up with an accurate number, you must include every measurement in your calculations.

In most cases, the cause of hypertension is unknown. The kidneys play an important role in controlling blood pressure, and the level of squeezing tension in the blood vessels makes a large contribution as well.

Lifestyle changes can dramatically reduce blood pressure. Increasing exercise, not smoking, and losing weight can all be highly effective. For many years doctors advised patients with hypertension to cut down on salt in the diet. Today, however, the value of this difficult dietary change has undergone significant questioning. Considering how rapidly our knowledge is evolving, I suggest consulting your physician to find the latest recommendations.

If lifestyle changes fail to reduce blood pressure, or if you can't make these alterations, many effective drugs are available. Sometimes you need to experiment with a few to find one that agrees with you.

Principal Natural Treatments for Hypertension

Although there are no well-documented natural treatments for hypertension, garlic and coenzyme Q_{10} have some evidence behind them and are reportedly quite effective. Keep in mind that when blood pressure is consistently higher than 160/110, nondrug treatments (other than lifestyle changes) are seldom enough to bring it down.

Garlic: Appears to Reduce Blood Pressure by 5 to 10%

At least 12 studies have examined garlic's effects on blood pressure, although only two of these involved people with hypertension.[1] Overall, it appears that garlic can reduce blood pressure levels by about 5 to 10%.

One of the best of these trials followed 47 subjects with average blood pressures of 171/101.[2] Over a period of 12 weeks, half were given placebo and the other half received 600 mg of garlic powder daily, standardized to 1.3% alliin. This is the most common form of medicinal garlic powder and is used for lowering cholesterol as well.

Compared to the placebo group, garlic reduced systolic blood pressure by 6% and diastolic pressure by 9%. Although this is not a dramatic improvement, it can definitely be useful.

A typical dosage of garlic is 900 mg daily of a garlic powder extract standardized to contain 1.3% alliin, providing about 12,000 mcg of alliin daily. Garlic is generally regarded as safe; however, because it appears to thin the blood it should not be combined with prescription anticoagulants, such as Coumadin (warfarin) or Trental (pentoxifylline). It also might not be a good idea to take garlic in the weeks before or after surgery or labor and delivery, or combine it with blood-thinning natural supplements such as ginkgo or high-dose vitamin E. (For more information on garlic, see the discussion under Cholesterol.)

Coenzyme Q$_{10}$: Appears Effective, but Needs More Study

The supplement coenzyme Q$_{10}$ (CoQ$_{10}$) is commonly recommended as a treatment for high blood pressure. One preliminary double-blind study found that 100 mg of CoQ_{10} daily reduced blood pressure by about the same amount as garlic.[3]

The usual dosage of CoQ_{10} is 30 to 100 mg 3 times daily. This supplement appears to be very safe. (For a more complete description of CoQ_{10}, see the discussion under Congestive Heart Failure.)

Other Natural Treatments for Hypertension

A number of other herbs and supplements may also be somewhat helpful for hypertension.

Fish Oil

Fish oil, a source of omega-3 fatty acids, is also commonly described as beneficial in the treatment of hypertension. However, the research record is mixed, and at best shows a slight benefit.[4] A typical dosage is 10 g daily. Fish oil frequently causes unpleasant burping. (See Essential Fatty Acids under Atherosclerosis for more information.)

Minerals: May Be Effective in Case of Deficiency

Adequate intake of calcium, magnesium, and potassium is necessary for good blood pressure control. When your body lacks adequate amounts of these minerals, supplementation may improve blood pressure.[5–12] However, in the absence of a deficiency, supplementation with these minerals probably will not produce any effect.

A dosage of 750 mg daily of calcium and 300 mg daily of supplemental magnesium should suffice. Individuals with severe kidney or heart disease should not take these otherwise safe supplements without consulting a physician, and if you have cancer, hyperparathyroidism, or sarcoidosis, you should not take calcium except on the advice of a physician. The best source of potassium is fruits and vegetables.

Hawthorn

The herb hawthorn is often said to reduce blood pressure, but there is no evidence that this is the case.[13] (For more information on hawthorn use and safety issues, see Congestive Heart Failure.)

Vitamin C: Probably Not Effective

Several studies suggest that vitamin C at a dosage of 1,000 mg or more taken daily may modestly reduce blood pressure.[14–17] However, none of these was double-blind. Strange as it may seem, the power of suggestion is quite capable of lowering blood pressure. When a double-blind study performed to evaluate the possible effectiveness of vitamin C found benefits, it found equal benefits in the placebo group as well.[18]

Other Treatments

Because atherosclerosis is the main harm caused by hypertension, treatments listed in Atherosclerosis should be considered as well.

IMPOTENCE

Principal Natural Treatments

There are no well-established natural treatments for impotence.

Other Natural Treatments

Ginkgo, ginseng, ashwaganda, suma, damiana, muira puama, zinc, L-arginine

Not Recommended Treatments

Yohimbe

Impotence, or erectile dysfunction, is the inability to achieve an erection. Impotence may occur for any of at least 15 possible causes, including diabetes, drug side effects, pituitary tumors, hardening of the arteries, hormonal imbalances, and psychological factors. A few of these conditions respond to specific treatment. For example, if a blood pressure drug is causing impotence, the best approach is to change drugs. If a pituitary tumor is secreting the hormone prolactin, treating that tumor may result in immediate improvement. However, in most cases, conventional treatment of impotence is nonspecific.

Generic treatment options include the drug Viagra, mechanical devices that utilize a vacuum to produce an erection, drugs for self-injection, and implantation of penile prostheses. Psychotherapy can also be helpful for treating all varieties of impotence, even when an organic cause can be identified.

Natural Treatments for Impotence

The following natural treatments are widely recommended for impotence, but they have not been scientifically proven effective at this time.

Ginkgo

A slight amount of research suggests that ginkgo may be useful in impotence. One study of 60 men whose impotence was due to poor blood circulation demonstrated a 50% success rate after 6 months.[1] However, because this was not a double-blind study, the improvement noted may have been due to the power of suggestion.

Recent reports suggest that ginkgo may also be useful in reversing the impotence caused by antidepressant drugs in the Prozac family.[2] (For more information on ginkgo, see the discussion under Alzheimer's Disease.)

Other Herbs

The herb yohimbe is the source of the drug yohimbine, which has been shown to be modestly better than placebo for impotence. However, this is a fairly dangerous treatment, and I do not recommend it.

Many other herbs are also reputed to improve sexual function, including ginseng, ashwaganda, suma, damiana, and muira puama.

Zinc

Zinc deficiency is known to negatively affect sexual function. Because zinc is one of the most commonly deficient minerals in the diet, it is logical to assume that supplementation with zinc may be helpful for some men. A typical dosage is 30 mg daily, taken with 1 to 2 mg of copper as supplemental zinc interferes with copper absorption. Too much zinc can be toxic, so do not exceed this dose.

L-Arginine

On the basis of minimal evidence, supplementation with L-arginine has also been recommended as a treatment for impotence. The usual dosage is 4 g daily, but the safety of L-arginine at this level is not known. However, because arginine restriction is often used to treat herpes, treatment with L-arginine might have the reverse effect (see the discussion of arginine and L-lysine under Herpes).

INFERTILITY IN MEN

Principal Natural Treatments
There are no well-established natural treatments for infertility in men.

Other Natural Treatments
Vitamin B_{12}, zinc, antioxidants (vitamin E, vitamin C), L-carnitine, beta-carotene, coenzyme Q_{10}, L-arginine, selenium

Male infertility, the inability of a man to produce a pregnancy in a woman, can be caused by a great variety of problems, from anatomical defects to hormonal imbalances. In about half of all cases, however, the source of the problem is never discovered.

The good news is that without any treatment at all, about 25% of supposedly infertile men bring about a pregnancy within a year of the time they first visit a physician for treatment. In other words, infertility is often only low fertility in disguise.

Natural Treatments for Male Infertility

The following natural treatments are widely recommended for male infertility, but they have not been scientifically proven effective at this time.

Vitamin B_{12}

Deficiencies in vitamin B_{12} lead to reduced sperm counts and lowered sperm mobility. Thus vitamin B_{12} supplementation might be expected to improve fertility in men who suffer from a deficiency of this essential vitamin. Mild B_{12} deficiencies are relatively common in people over 60.[1]

A couple of preliminary studies suggest that B_{12} supplementation (1,000 mcg daily) can sometimes improve sperm counts and sperm activity even when no deficiency exists.[2,3] Unfortunately, improving sperm counts and mobility does not necessarily translate into increased fertility (although it wouldn't hurt). Vitamin B_{12} is believed to be extremely safe.

Zinc

Zinc is also an essential nutrient for proper sperm production, and deficiency may result in lowered testosterone levels.[4] One preliminary study found not only an increase in sperm counts, but also an actual increase in pregnancy rate when men with low testosterone were given zinc supplements.[5] However, those whose testosterone levels were normal did not benefit. The proper dosage of zinc is about 30 mg daily, coupled with 1 mg of copper for balance. Too much zinc can be toxic, so do not exceed this dose.

Antioxidants

Free radicals, dangerous chemicals found naturally in the body, may damage sperm. For this reason, a number of studies have evaluated the benefits of antioxidants for male infertility.

In one placebo-controlled study of 52 men whose sperm showed subnormal activity, daily treatment with 100 IU of vitamin E resulted in improved sperm activity and increased rate of pregnancy in their partners.[6] (For more information and safety issues, see the discussion of vitamin E in Atherosclerosis.)

Preliminary studies suggest that vitamin C may also help.[7] The higher the dose of the vitamin, the quicker the benefit starts; but even low doses produce good results given time. The dosages studied ranged from 200 to 1,000 mg daily. (For a discussion of safety issues involving vitamin C, see the discussion under Cataracts.)

Other Supplements

Many other supplements have been suggested as treatments for infertility, including L-carnitine, beta-carotene, coenzyme Q_{10}, L-arginine, and selenium. However, the evidence that they really work is negligible, and studies on the last two supplements have shown more negative than positive results.

All the treatments listed in Impotence have also been proposed as treatments for male infertility.

INFERTILITY IN WOMEN

Principal Natural Treatments
There are no well-established natural treatments for
infertility in women.

Other Natural Treatments
Chasteberry, multivitamins

There are many possible causes of female infertility. Tubal
disease and endometriosis (a condition in which uterine
tissue begins to grow where it shouldn't) account for 50%
of female infertility; failure of ovulation is the cause of
about 30%; and cervical factors cause another 10%.

An immense industry has sprung up around correcting
female infertility, using techniques that range from hormone therapy to in vitro (test-tube) babies. Although
these methods have their occasional stunning successes,
there is considerable controversy about the high cost and
low rate of effectiveness of fertility treatments in general.
The good news is that apparently infertile women often
eventually become pregnant with no medical intervention
at all.

Natural Treatments for Female Infertility
The following natural treatments are widely recommended for female infertility, but they have not been scientifically proven effective at this time.

Chasteberry
The herb chasteberry is widely used in Europe as a treatment for infertility.[1] It is believed to work by reducing excessive levels of prolactin, a hormone produced by the
pituitary gland.

The typical dose of chasteberry extract is 20 to 40 mg given once a day. Chasteberry is sold often as a liquid extract to be taken at a dosage of 40 drops each morning. However, highly concentrated extracts are also available that require much lower dosing. Chasteberry's safety has not been adequately evaluated. (See PMS for a further discussion of chasteberry use and safety issues.)

Multivitamins

According to one study, general supplementation with multivitamins may improve female fertility.[2]

INSOMNIA

Principal Natural Treatments
Valerian, melatonin

Other Natural Treatments
Kava, hops, passionflower, skullcap, lady's slipper,
St. John's wort, 5-hydroxytryptophan

According to recent reports, many people today have a serious problem getting a good night's sleep. Our lives are simply too busy for us to get the 8 hours we really need. To make matters worse, many of us suffer from insomnia. When we do get to bed, we may stay awake thinking for hours. Sleep itself may be restless instead of refreshing.

Most people who sleep substantially less than 8 hours a night experience a variety of unpleasant symptoms. The most common are headaches, mental confusion, irritability, malaise, immune deficiencies, depression, and fatigue. Complete sleep deprivation can lead to hallucinations and mental collapse.

The best ways to improve sleep are lifestyle changes: eliminating caffeine and sugar from your diet, avoiding stimulating activities before bed, adopting a regular sleeping time, and gradually turning down the lights.

Many drugs can also help with sleep. Such medications as Ambien, Restoril, Ativan, Valium, Xanax, and chloral hydrate are widely used for sleep problems. However, these medications tend to promote tolerance and dependency on the drug, and can even cause addiction.

Recently, physicians have come to regard some forms of insomnia as a variation of depression. This conclusion comes from a kind of reverse reasoning: We know that depression almost always disturbs sleep, and that antidepressants frequently help insomnia. Therefore, maybe some cases of insomnia really are depression in disguise.

Antidepressants can be used in two ways to correct sleep problems. Low doses of certain antidepressants immediately bring on sleep because their side effects include drowsiness. However, this effect tends to wear off with repeated use.

For chronic sleeping problems, full doses of antidepressants may be necessary. Antidepressants are believed to work by actually altering brain chemistry, which produces a beneficial effect on sleep. Trazodone and Serzone are two of the most commonly prescribed antidepressants when improved sleep is desired, but most other antidepressants can be helpful as well.

Principal Natural Treatments for Insomnia

Although the scientific evidence isn't yet definitive, the herb valerian and the hormone melatonin are widely accepted as treatments for certain forms of insomnia.

Valerian: Appears to Improve Sleep Gradually

Over 200 plant species belong to the genus *Valeriana,* but the species used for insomnia is *Valeriana officinalis.* This perennial grows abundantly in moist woodlands in Europe and North America and is under extensive cultivation to meet market demands. The root is used for medicinal purposes.

Valerian has a long traditional use for insomnia. Galen recommended valerian for insomnia in the second century A.D. The herb became popular in Europe from the sixteenth century onward as a sedative, and was widely used in the United States as well until the 1950s. Rumors have it that Valium was named to imitate the sound of valerian, although there is no chemical similarity between the two.

Proper scientific studies of valerian did not begin until the 1980s. The results ultimately led to its approval by Germany's Commission E in 1985. Presently, valerian is an accepted over-the-counter drug for insomnia in Germany, Belgium, France, Switzerland, and Italy.

Valerian is commonly recommended as an aid for occasional insomnia. However, the results of a recent study suggest that it may be more useful for long-term improvement of sleep.[1]

What Is the Scientific Evidence for Valerian?

Constituents of valerian as well as whole-valerian extracts have been shown to act as sedatives in laboratory animals.[2,3,4] Studies in humans have also found that valerian is an effective sleeping aid.

A recent 28-day, double-blind placebo-controlled study followed 121 people with histories of significant sleep disturbance.[5] This study looked at the effectiveness of 600 mg of an alcohol-based valerian extract taken 2 hours before bedtime.

Valerian didn't work right away. For the first couple of weeks, valerian and placebo were running neck and neck. However, by day 28 valerian had pulled far ahead. Effectiveness was rated as good or very good by participant evaluation in 66% of the valerian group and in 61% by doctor evaluation, whereas in the placebo group, only

29% were so rated by participants and doctors. Only two individuals reported side effects, which were mild.

This study provides good evidence that valerian is effective for insomnia. However, it has one confusing aspect: the 4-week delay before effects were seen. In previous smaller studies, valerian has produced an immediately noticeable effect on sleep,[6–9] and that is what most practitioners believe to be typical. Why valerian took so long to work in this one study has not been explained.

We don't really know how valerian acts to induce sleep. Research suggests that the neurotransmitter GABA may be involved.[10–16] Conventional sleeping pills affect GABA as well.

Dosage

For insomnia, the standard dosage of valerian is 2 to 3 g dried root, 270 to 450 mg of a water-based valerian extract (3–6:1), or 600 mg of an alcohol-based extract (4–7:1) taken 1 to 2 hours before bedtime.[17] If the results of the most recent study are correct, 4 weeks of continuous treatment may be necessary to achieve full results.

Safety Issues

Valerian is listed on the FDA's "generally regarded as safe" (GRAS) list and is approved for use as a food. Overdoses as high as 20 times the normal dose have not been associated with significant problems.[18] Very high doses have been given to rats without ill effects.[19]

Except for the unpleasant odor, valerian generally produces few to no side effects. In a study of 61 individuals taking normal doses of valerian, only 2 people reported side effects, which consisted of headache and morning grogginess.[20] Mild gastrointestinal distress is also occasionally reported, and, strangely, a few people experience a mild stimulant effect from valerian.

Valerian does not appear to impair driving ability or cause morning grogginess when taken at night.[21,22]

However, it can impair alertness for a couple of hours immediately after use. For this reason, driving a car or operating hazardous machinery immediately after taking valerian is not recommended. According to the results of one animal study, valerian should not be combined with other medications that might make you drowsy.[23] However, a study in 1995 found no interaction between alcohol and valerian as measured by concentration, attentiveness, reaction time, and driving performance.[24]

Addiction to valerian has not been observed in studies. However, at the time of this writing there has been a disturbing report of severe withdrawal symptoms in a man who took valerian for many months and then stopped suddenly. This potentially serious problem needs urgent investigation.

The safety of valerian for young children, pregnant or nursing women, and those with liver or kidney disease has not been established.

Melatonin: Rapid Effect on Sleep

The body uses melatonin as part of its normal control of the sleep-wake cycle. The pineal gland makes serotonin and then turns it into melatonin when exposure to light decreases. Strong light (such as sunlight) slows melatonin production more than weak light does, and a completely dark room increases the amount of melatonin made more than a partially darkened room does.[25]

Taking melatonin as a supplement seems to stimulate sleep when the natural cycle is disturbed. It is most dramatically effective for jet lag and for those who work the night shift and want to change sleeping time on the weekends.

What Is the Scientific Evidence for Melatonin?

One double-blind study tracked 320 people who were given 5 mg of standard melatonin, 5 mg of slow-release melatonin, 0.5 mg of standard melatonin, or placebo for 4 nights following plane travel.[26] The results showed improvements only with 5 mg of standard melatonin. Benefits were noted in quality of sleep, the time needed to fall asleep, and daytime drowsiness and fatigue.

Positive results were seen in several other studies,[27,28,29] although at least one negative study has been reported.[30]

According to one review of the literature, treatment is most effective for those who have crossed more than eight time zones.[31] However, melatonin also seems to help bring on sleep for other people, including those with no sleep problems to begin with.

Dosage

Melatonin is typically taken about 30 to 60 minutes before bedtime during the first 4 days after traveling.

The ideal dosage of melatonin is not known. According to some reports, 0.5 mg is the minimum effective dose. However, one study described above found no effect at 0.5 mg but good results at 5 mg.[32] To further complicate matters, this study also found that only quick-release melatonin was effective, while in other studies time-release forms have proved more effective. Clearly, there is much we do not know about melatonin.

Safety Issues

Melatonin is probably safe for occasional use (as in plane travel), but there is some real concern about using it on a regular basis. Keep in mind that melatonin is not really a food supplement: It is a hormone, just like estrogen, thyroid, or cortisone. Because the body's own production of melatonin is probably the equivalent of a dosage of only 0.1 mg daily, when you take melatonin for sleep you are tremendously exceeding natural levels. The consequences of doing so on a regular basis are completely unknown.[33]

Based on theoretical ideas of how melatonin works, some authorities specifically recommend against its use in depression, schizophrenia, autoimmune diseases, and other serious illnesses and for pregnant or nursing women. Do not drive or operate machinery for several hours after taking melatonin.

Other Natural Treatments for Insomnia

The following natural treatments are widely recommended for insomnia, but they have not been scientifically proven effective at this time.

Kava

The antianxiety herb kava is also said to be helpful for insomnia. A typical dose of standardized extract should provide about 180 to 210 mg of kavalactones and should be taken 1 hour before bedtime. (For more information on kava use and safety issues, see the discussion under Anxiety.)

Other Herbal Sedatives

Many other herbs are famous for their sedative properties, including hops, passionflower, skullcap, and lady's slipper. However, there has been little to no scientific evaluation of the safety or effectiveness of these herbs.

St. John's Wort

Because prescription antidepressants can help you sleep, it has been suggested that the herb St. John's wort may be useful in the same way.

St. John's wort does not cause immediate drowsiness like some pharmaceutical antidepressants. Rather, if it is effective, the results will develop gradually. (For more information on St. John's wort, see the discussion under Depression.)

Tryptophan and 5-Hydroxytryptophan

For many years, people used tryptophan as a sleeping aid. However, an accidental poisonous contaminant in one batch caused many cases of a terrible illness called eosinophilic myalgia. Tryptophan has since been taken off the shelves.

The substance 5-hydroxytryptophan (5-HTP) has recently become widely available as a substitute. Because it is made by a completely different manufacturing process (starting from a plant rather than a bacteria), one would not expect the same contaminant to appear. Surprisingly, however, in September 1998 the FDA released a report stating that there was some evidence that commercial 5-HTP preparations might contain a similar contaminant. Because this is late-breaking news, I suggest you check with your physician for the most recent information.

A typical dosage is 100 to 300 mg at bedtime. (For more information on 5-HTP, see the discussion under Depression.)

INTERMITTENT CLAUDICATION
(Peripheral Vascular Disease)

Principal Natural Treatments
Ginkgo, L-carnitine

The arteries supplying the legs with blood may become seriously blocked in advanced stages of atherosclerosis (hardening of the arteries). This can lead to severe, crampy pain when you walk more than a short distance, because the muscles are starved for oxygen. In fact, the intensity of intermittent claudication is often measured in the distance a person can walk without pain.

Conventional treatment for intermittent claudication consists of measures to combat atherosclerosis, the drug Trental (pentoxifylline), and other medications. In advanced cases, surgery to improve blood flow may be necessary.

Principal Natural Treatments for Intermittent Claudication

A number of natural treatments may be helpful, but it isn't clear whether it is safe to combine them with the medications that may be prescribed at the same time. Medical supervision is definitely necessary for this serious disease.

Because they work so differently, it has been suggested that the two treatments described in this section, ginkgo and carnitine, might enhance each other's effectiveness when taken together.

Ginkgo

Germany's Commission E authorizes the use of ginkgo (described in more detail under Alzheimer's Disease) for the treatment of intermittent claudication. Several preliminary double-blind studies suggest that ginkgo can produce a significant increase in pain-free walking distance, probably by improving circulation.[1,2,3]

The most recent of these studies enrolled 111 patients and followed them for 24 weeks.[4] Subjects were measured for pain-free walking distance by walking up a 12% slope on a treadmill at 2 miles an hour. At the beginning of treatment, both the placebo and ginkgo groups were able to walk about 107 meters without pain.

At the end of the trial, both groups had improved significantly (the power of placebo is amazing!) However, the ginkgo group had improved more, reaching an average of 153 meters compared to 127 meters for the control group.

Bottom line: Ginkgo extract can reduce symptoms and produce measurable if not dramatic improvements in walking distance.

The typical dosage of ginkgo is 40 mg 3 times daily. Ginkgo generally does not cause side effects, but fears that it may interact with blood-thinning medications (see the discussion under Alzheimer's disease) make its use in intermittent claudication difficult. To safely use ginkgo, you may have to decline conventional treatment, and this could be a very risky decision.

L-Carnitine

The vitamin-like substance L-carnitine (discussed in more detail in Angina) also appears to be of some benefit in intermittent claudication. Although it does not increase blood flow, carnitine appears to increase walking distance by improving energy utilization in the muscles.

A recent double-blind study followed 245 people, half of whom were treated with a special form of L-carnitine called L-propionyl-carnitine, the other half took placebo.[5] A dosage of 2,000 mg daily produced an average 73% improvement in walking distance, compared to a 46% improvement in the placebo group. Reductions in pain levels were also reported.

The optimum dosage of L-propionyl-carnitine appears to be 1 to 2 g daily. This apparently safe supplement is not associated with any significant side effects, toxicities, or drug interactions. However, individuals on kidney dialysis should not use L-carnitine (or any other supplement) except on medical advice.

IRRITABLE BOWEL SYNDROME
(Spastic Colon)

Principal Natural Treatments
Peppermint oil

The symptoms of irritable bowel syndrome (IBS) include one or more of the following: alternating diarrhea and constipation, intestinal gas, bloating and cramping, abdominal pain, painful bowel movements, mucous discharge, and undigested food in the stool. Despite all these distressing symptoms, in IBS the intestines appear to be perfectly healthy when they are examined. Thus the condition belongs to a category of diseases that physicians call *functional.* This term means that while the function of the bowel seems to have gone awry, no injury or disturbance of its structure can be discovered.

The cause of IBS remains unknown. Medical treatment for irritable bowel syndrome consists mainly of increased dietary fiber plus drugs that reduce bowel spasm.

Principal Natural Treatments
for Irritable Bowel Syndrome

Peppermint oil is widely used for IBS. However, the research evidence is a bit contradictory.[1–4] The proper dosage is 1 or 2 capsules (0.2 ml per capsule) 3 times daily between meals. Because dosage amounts of peppermint needed to relieve lower bowel cramping can cause heartburn, the best formulations are specially enteric coated to pass intact through the stomach (this is usually stated on the label).

When taken as directed, peppermint is believed to be reasonably safe in healthy adults.[5] However, peppermint can cause jaundice in newborn babies, so do not try to use it for colic. Excessive intake of peppermint oil can cause nausea, loss of appetite, heart problems, loss of balance, and other nervous system problems.

Safety in pregnant or nursing women or those with severe liver or kidney disease has not been established.

MACULAR DEGENERATION

Principal Natural Treatments
Antioxidants (vitamin C, vitamin E, selenium, beta-carotene, lutein, zeaxanthin, lycopene, bilberry, ginkgo, grape seed, wine)
Other Natural Treatments
Zinc

The lens of the eye focuses an image of the world on a portion of the retina called the *macula*, the area of finest visual perception. After cataracts, damage to the macula is the second most common cause of visual impairment in those over 65. Smoking, high blood pressure, and atherosclerosis are associated with macular degeneration. Bright light also appears to play a role by creating damaging natural substances in the eye, called free radicals. Gradual deterioration of the macula is called macular degeneration.

In the most common form of macular degeneration, a substance known as lipofuscin accumulates in the lining of the retina. No conventional medical treatment is available for this disease, although mainstream researchers are seriously investigating the antioxidants described here.

A much less common form of macular degeneration involves the abnormal growth of blood vessels. This can be treated very successfully, if attended to soon enough, but may lead to irreversible blindness if left untreated. For this reason, medical consultation in all cases of macular degeneration (or any other type of vision loss) is essential.

Principal Natural Treatments for Macular Degeneration

Because research suggests that macular degeneration may be related to free radical damage, it's natural to reason that antioxidant nutrients may be able to protect against it. However, more research is necessary for firm conclusions.

An observational study of 2,152 subjects, aged 43 to 86, found that vitamin C supplementation was associated with a decreased incidence of early age-related macular degeneration.[1] Another observational study enrolling almost 2,000 people found that high intake of vitamin C or E was associated with less macular degeneration.[2]

It may be that combinations of many antioxidants, such as those found in foods, are most beneficial. One 18-month, double-blind study found that a daily supplement containing 750 mg vitamin C, 200 IU vitamin E, 50 mcg selenium, and 20,000 IU beta-carotene stopped progression of macular degeneration.[3] (For more information and safety issues for vitamin C, see the discussion under Cataracts. Vitamin E is discussed at length under Atherosclerosis, and selenium is discussed under Cancer.)

Various dietary carotenes may also be associated with a lower incidence of macular degeneration.[4,5] Carotenes (carotenoids) are a group of substances that are found in many fruits and vegetables, especially yellow-orange and dark-green ones. Beta-carotene is the most famous carotene. However, the less well known carotenes lutein and zeaxanthin may be more closely correlated with protection from macular degeneration. These are principally found in dark-green leafy vegetables, such as spinach and collard greens. It has been suggested that lutein may protect the macula from light-induced damage by dying it yellow, thereby acting as a kind of natural sunglasses.[6] It also acts in the usual antioxidant fashion by neutralizing free radicals.[7] Lycopene, a carotenoid found in tomatoes, may also be helpful.

Flavonoids are another group of naturally occurring chemicals, found in many plants, that may offer a variety of beneficial effects. Weak but interesting evidence suggests that the flavonoid-rich herbs bilberry, ginkgo, and grape seed may prevent or treat macular degeneration.[8,9,10] (For more information, see *The Natural Pharmacist: Your Complete Guide to Herbs.*)

Moderate wine consumption appears to help prevent macular degeneration.[11] Like these herbs, wine contains high levels of flavonoids.

Other Natural Treatments for Macular Degeneration

The mineral zinc may also help prevent macular degeneration, although the study results are a bit contradictory.[12,13,14] A typical dosage is 15 to 30 mg daily, combined with 1 to 3 mg of copper to avoid zinc-induced copper deficiency. Too much zinc can be toxic, so do not exceed this dose.

MENOPAUSAL SYMPTOMS
(Other Than Osteoporosis)

Principal Natural Treatments

Black cohosh, soy isoflavones

Other Natural Treatments

Vitamin E, vitamin C, bioflavonoids, essential fatty acids, rice bran extract, licorice, chasteberry, dong quai

The hormonal changes of menopause can produce a wide variety of symptoms, ranging from hot flashes and vaginal dryness to anxiety, depression, and insomnia. Many of these symptoms are undoubtedly caused by the natural decrease in estrogen production that occurs at menopause;

however, the human body is so complex that other hormonal factors also play a role.

Menopause is not a disease. It is clearly a natural process, but one that has fallen out of favor in modern society. We no longer consider it as an inevitable transition, but instead treat it as a condition requiring treatment. No longer do women accept as merely part of life the decrease in libido, pain during intercourse, years of hot flashes, and other uncomfortable problems that may accompany menopause. This raises an important point: How close to nature do we want to live? One of the most valued ideals of alternative medicine is the desire to trust nature, but sometimes we may want to draw a line. For example, in a state of nature, infant and maternal mortality is high. This process of survival of the fittest helps humanity as a species to be stronger, but it is not something that a compassionate society can tolerate. Thus, no matter what our ideals, we frequently find ourselves tampering with nature. The treatment of menopause is simply one example among many.

Conventional medicine recommends the use of replacement estrogen to provide three benefits: eliminating the symptoms of menopause, protecting against osteoporosis, and maintaining the protection against cardiovascular disease that premenopausal women enjoy.

Estrogen-replacement therapy is quite effective at achieving these goals. However, like most medical treatments, it creates counterbalancing risks. The most frightening issue is the increased risk of breast cancer that appears to be associated with replacement estrogen. The decision whether to use estrogen-replacement therapy should involve a careful examination of the risks and benefits in consultation with a physician. Specially modified estrogens, such as Evista (raloxifene), appear to help osteoporosis and reduce the incidence of breast cancer, but they do not reduce symptoms of menopause.

Principal Natural Treatments for Menopausal Symptoms

Several natural treatments may reduce menopausal symptoms. However, we do not know for sure whether any of these reduce the risk of cardiovascular disease or osteoporosis. (See Atherosclerosis and Osteoporosis for natural ways to reduce the risk of these conditions.)

Black Cohosh: Widely Used in Europe for Menopausal Symptoms

Black cohosh is a tall perennial herb that was originally found in the northeastern United States. Native Americans used it mainly for women's health problems but also as a treatment for arthritis, fatigue, and snakebite. European colonists rapidly adopted the herb for similar uses.

In the late nineteenth century, black cohosh was the main ingredient in the wildly popular Lydia E. Pinkham's Vegetable Compound for menstrual cramps. Migrating across the Atlantic, black cohosh became a popular European treatment for women's problems, arthritis, and high blood pressure. In the 1980s, black cohosh was approved by Germany's Commission E for use in menopause.

What Is the Scientific Evidence for Black Cohosh?

Evidence suggests that over a period of 4 to 6 weeks black cohosh can improve all major menopausal symptoms, including hot flashes, sweating, headache, vertigo, heart palpitations, tinnitus, nervousness, irritability, sleep disturbance, anxiety, vaginal dryness, and depression.[1,2,3] Unfortunately, there is no evidence that black cohosh can prevent osteoporosis or heart disease, two of estrogen's most famous benefits.

A double-blind study of 80 participants compared the benefits of black cohosh, estrogen (0.625 mg), and placebo over a period of 12 weeks.[4] Black cohosh proved at least as effective as estrogen in reducing all the major symptoms of menopause. It also helped reverse the menopause-related changes in vaginal cells. Similar results were seen in other studies.[5,6]

Black cohosh is made up of many substances called phytoestrogens, which have shown some estrogen-like activity in test-tube studies. Extracts of the herb reduce levels of the pituitary hormone LH (luteinizing hormone), just like standard estrogen-replacement therapy.[7,8,9] Thus, up until 1998 it was believed that black cohosh worked by imitating some of the effects of estrogen.

However, matters were recently made more complicated when an unpublished, double-blind study reported in the product literature of one manufacturer of black cohosh found no evidence of improvement in vaginal cells or other evidence of estrogen-like activity.[10] This surprising finding has upset the apple cart, leaving us quite confused today regarding just how black cohosh really works.

Dosage

The standard dosage of black cohosh is 1 to 2 tablets twice daily of a standardized extract manufactured to contain 1 mg of 27-deoxyacteine per tablet.

Make sure not to confuse black cohosh with blue cohosh (*Caulophyllum thalictroides*). Blue cohosh is potentially more dangerous because it contains chemicals that are toxic to the heart. A recent case report indicates that it caused severe heart problems in a woman who took blue cohosh during pregnancy.[11]

Safety Issues

Black cohosh seldom produces any obvious side effects, other than occasional mild gastrointestinal distress. Studies in rats have shown no significant toxicity when black cohosh was given at 90 times the therapeutic dosage for a period of 6 months.[12] Because 6 months in a rat corresponds to decades in a human, this study appears to make a strong statement about the long-term safety of black cohosh.

Unlike estrogen, black cohosh does not stimulate breast cancer cells growing in a test tube, probably because the estrogens it contains are weaker than human estrogen.[13] However, this should not be taken as a guarantee that black cohosh does not increase the risk of breast cancer. Women who have already had breast cancer should not take black cohosh except on the advice of a physician.

Black cohosh has been shown to slightly lower blood pressure and blood sugar in certain animals.[14] For this reason, it's possible that the herb could interact with drugs for high blood pressure or diabetes, although no such problems have been reported.

Black cohosh is generally not recommended for pregnant or nursing mothers, and safety in young children and those with severe liver or kidney disease has not been established.

Soy Isoflavones: May Reduce Symptoms

Black cohosh isn't the only plant that contains estrogen-like substances. Soy also contains phytoestrogens called *isoflavones,* which appear to produce far-reaching effects in the body. The most famous of these isoflavones are genistein and daidzen. These substances, or their combination, appear to be effective in reducing menopausal hot flashes. In one double-blind study of 104 women, daily doses of 60 g of a soy product significantly reduced flushing associated with menopause.[15] However, soy does not appear to reduce vaginal dryness.

It is not known whether soy can prevent osteoporosis.[16] However, a synthetic isoflavone named ipriflavone (chemically similar to what is found in soy) does seem to be effective for this purpose. (See Osteoporosis for more information.)

Soy may be protective against heart disease and breast and uterine cancer, but this has not been definitively proven. However, soy may not be safe for those who have already had breast cancer.

The best dosage of soy is unclear. One or two cups of soy milk or slices of tofu daily appear to be helpful.[17]

Various products containing concentrated phytoestrogens from soy or red clover have recently come on the market. However, although these supplements show promise, more research needs to be done to establish the correct dosage and to verify safety.

Other Natural Treatments
for Menopausal Symptoms

Vitamin E, vitamin C, bioflavonoids, essential fatty acids, an extract of rice bran called gamma oryzanol, and the herbs licorice and chasteberry are reportedly helpful for menopause. However, there is little to no scientific evidence to turn to.

The herb dong quai is also frequently recommended for menopausal symptoms, but a recent double-blind study found it to be entirely ineffective.[18]

(For more information on menopause, see *The Natural Pharmacist Guide to Menopause.*)

MIGRAINE HEADACHES

Principal Natural Treatments
Feverfew, magnesium

Other Natural Treatments
5-hydroxytryptophan, fish oil, riboflavin, chromium, calcium, vitamin D, vitamin C, vitamin B_6, thiamine, folic acid, niacin, ginger, allergen-free diet, acupuncture

The term *migraine* refers to a class of headaches sharing certain characteristic symptoms. The two main subcategories of migraine are the common and the classic migraine.

In common migraines, headache pain usually occurs in the forehead or temples, often on one side only and typically accompanied by nausea and a preference for a darkened room. Headache attacks last for several hours up to a day or more. They are usually separated by completely pain-free intervals.

In the rarer form of migraine, called classic migraine, headache pain is accompanied by a visual disturbance known as an aura. Otherwise, symptoms are similar to those of the common migraine.

Migraines can be triggered by a variety of causes, including fatigue, stress, hormonal changes, and foods such as alcohol, chocolate, peanuts, and avocados. However, in many people, migraines occur with no obvious triggering factor.

The cause of migraine headaches has been a subject of continuing controversy for over a century. Opinion has swung back and forth between two primary beliefs: that migraines are related to epileptic seizures and originate in the nervous tissue of the brain; or that blood vessels in the skull cause headache pain when they dilate or contract (so-called vascular headaches). Most likely, several factors are involved, and more than one stimulus can light the fuse that leads to a full-blown migraine attack.

Conventional treatment of acute migraines has lately been revolutionized by the drug sumatriptan (Imitrex). This drug can completely abort a migraine headache in many individuals. It works by imitating the action of serotonin on blood vessels, causing them to contract. Drugs made from ergot mold are also effective.

People interested in prevention can choose from a bewildering variety of drugs, including ergot drugs, antidepressants, beta-blockers, calcium channel–blockers, and antiseizure medication. Picking the right one is mostly a matter of trial and error.

(For more information on migraine headaches, see *The Natural Pharmacist Guide to Feverfew and Migraines.*)

Principal Natural Treatments for Migraine Headaches

Scientific evidence suggests that the herb feverfew and the mineral magnesium can help prevent migraine headaches.

Keep in mind that serious diseases may occasionally first present themselves as migraine-type headaches. If you suddenly start having migraines without a previous history, or if the pattern of your migraines changes significantly, it is essential to seek medical evaluation.

Feverfew: Dried Leaf May Reduce Frequency and Severity of Headaches

Feverfew was widely used in ancient times as a treatment for headaches and other conditions. However, it fell out of favor for several centuries, until an unexpected but fortunate event occurred in the late 1970s. At that time, the wife of the chief medical officer of the National Coal Board in England suffered from serious migraine headaches. When this fact became known to workers in the industry, a sympathetic miner suggested that she try a folk treatment he knew about. She followed his advice and chewed feverfew leaves. The results were dramatic: Her migraines almost completely disappeared.

Her husband was impressed, too, and used his high office to gain the ear of a physician who specialized in migraine headaches, Dr. E. Stewart Johnson of the London

Migraine Clinic. Johnson subsequently tried feverfew on 10 of his patients. The results were so good that he subsequently gave the herb to 270 of his patients. A whopping 70% reported considerable relief.

Thoroughly excited now, Dr. Johnson enrolled 17 feverfew-using patients in an interesting type of double-blind study.[1] Half were continued on feverfew, and the other half transferred without their knowledge to placebo. Over a period of 6 months, the participants withdrawn from feverfew demonstrated a dramatic increase in headaches, nausea, and vomiting.

Unfortunately, this study had some serious flaws. It was too small, and because the participants were already feverfew users who felt it worked for them, it didn't say anything about the effectiveness of feverfew in the population at large. This type of error in a study is called *self-selection*. Nonetheless, the study brought a flood of response from the public and ultimately led to three preliminary but properly performed double-blind experiments.

Today, feverfew is used mainly for the prevention of chronic, recurrent migraine headaches, especially in the United Kingdom. Those who use it say that their headaches become less frequent and less severe, and may even stop altogether. However, feverfew must be taken religiously every day for best results.

Reportedly, feverfew taken at the onset of a migraine attack can provide some benefit, but no studies have yet been performed to confirm this. It is not at all effective for cluster or tension headaches.

What Is the Scientific Evidence for Feverfew?

Two double-blind studies suggest that regular use of feverfew leaf can help prevent migraine headaches and reduce their severity when they do come.

The so-called Nottingham trial followed 59 individuals for 8 months.[2] For 4 months, half received a daily capsule of feverfew leaf, and the other half received placebo. The groups were then switched and followed for an additional 4 months. Treatment with feverfew produced a 24% reduction in the number of migraines and a significant decrease in nausea and vomiting during the headaches.

A recent double-blind study of 57 people with migraines, who were given feverfew leaf daily, also showed distinct reductions in headache severity.[3] Unfortunately, the authors did not report whether the frequency of headaches improved.

However, the herb world was surprised when a Dutch study of 50 people showed no difference whatsoever between placebo and a special feverfew extract standardized to its parthenolide content.[4] This unexpected result reversed a widely held view about how feverfew works.

For many years it was assumed that the active ingredient in feverfew was a substance named parthenolide. Many articles were published explaining exactly how parthenolide prevented migraines.[5–8] On the basis of this premature explanation, indignant authors complained that samples of feverfew on the market vary as much as 10 to 1 in their parthenolide content. No less an authority than the herbal expert Varro Tyler said that "standardization of the herbal material on the basis of its parthenolide content is urgently required if this potentially valuable herb is to be used effectively." [9]

However, everyone was jumping the gun. The special feverfew extract used in the negative Dutch study was standardized to a high parthenolide content. Apparently, this extract lacked some essential substance or group of substances that is present in the whole leaf, which was used in the positive studies. Without these unknown constituents, it seems that feverfew does not work. What those substances may have been remains mysterious.

Dosage

The daily dosage of feverfew used in the Nottingham study was 82 mg of dried leaf containing 0.66% parthenolide. Subsequent dosage recommendations tended to concentrate on reproducing about the same daily quantity of parthenolide. However, now that the importance of parthenolide has been cast in doubt, it is no longer clear what sources of feverfew are effective or at what precise dosage they should be taken. It is probably safe to say that at the present time dried whole leaf is a better bet than feverfew extract.

Safety Issues

Among the many thousands of people who use feverfew as a folk medicine in England, no reports of serious toxicity have been published.

In the 8-month Nottingham clinical trial of 76 participants (59 completed the study), no significant differences in side effects were found between treated individuals and the placebo group, nor were any changes in measurements on blood tests and urinalysis noted.[10]

In a survey of 300 study participants, 11.3% reported mouth sores after chewing feverfew leaf, occasionally accompanied by general inflammation of tissues in the mouth.[11] A smaller percentage reported mild gastrointestinal distress.[12] However, mouth sores do not seem to occur in people who use encapsulated feverfew.

Animal studies confirm the safety of feverfew. No adverse effects were seen at doses 100 and 150 times the human daily dose in rats and guinea pigs respectively.[13]

However, because feverfew was an old folk remedy used to promote abortions, it should probably not be taken during pregnancy. Safety in young children and those with severe liver or kidney disease has also not been established.

Magnesium: May Help Prevent Migraines

Magnesium is another natural treatment that appears to be effective for the prevention of migraine headaches. A recent 12-week double-blind study followed 81 people with recurrent migraines.[14] Half received 600 mg of magnesium daily (in the rather unusual form of trimagnesium dicitrate), and the other half received placebo.

By the last 3 weeks of the study, the frequency of migraine attacks was reduced by 41.6% in the treated group, compared to 15.8% in the placebo group. The only side effects observed were diarrhea (18.6%) and digestive irritation (4.7%).

Similar results have been seen in other double-blind studies.[15,16] There was one study that did not find a benefit,[17] but there were many problems with its design.[18]

Since many people are deficient in magnesium anyway, it's hard to go wrong taking a magnesium supplement. The usual nutritional dose is in the neighborhood of 350 mg daily, but 600 mg (as used in the study) should be safe, unless you suffer from severe heart or kidney disease.

Other Natural Treatments for Migraine Headaches

Several other herbs and supplements are widely recommended for migraine headaches, but as yet there is little scientific proof that they are effective.

5-Hydroxytryptophan

The supplement 5-hydroxytryptophan (5-HTP) has also been suggested as a treatment for migraine headaches. (See the longer discussion of this supplement under Depression.) However, the available scientific evidence is contradictory at best.

The body manufactures 5-HTP on the way to making serotonin. It is possible, but not yet proven, that supplemental 5-HTP may increase serotonin levels. Serotonin is believed to be involved in the beginning of migraine headaches, and, as described previously, the dramatically effective antimigraine drug Imitrex works by imitating the effects of serotonin on blood vessels. Antidepressants that appear to raise serotonin levels in general, such as Prozac, sometimes seem to help prevent migraines as well. 5-HTP may provide similar benefits.

One study compared the effectiveness of 5-HTP against the standard migraine drug methysergide. In this 6-month trial of 124 participants, 5-HTP proved to be equally effective.[19] Benefits were more dramatic in the strength and duration than in the frequency of attacks. Because methysergide has been proven to be better than placebo, the study results provide meaningful, although not airtight, evidence that 5-HTP is effective as well.

However, in a double-blind study that directly compared 5-HTP to placebo, 5-HTP failed to produce significantly better results than the placebo.[20] And in another study, 5-HTP was not as effective as the drug propranolol.[21] A few studies have found benefits for children and adolescents with various types of headaches, including migraines.[22,23]

Putting all this information together, it appears that 5-HTP is possibly an effective treatment for the prevention of migraines. (There are some safety concerns regarding 5-HTP. See the discussion under Depression.)

Fish Oil

Preliminary double-blind studies suggest that high doses of fish oil may be helpful for migraine headaches.[24,25] (See Essential Fatty Acids under Atherosclerosis for further discussion of fish oil.)

Other Supplements

Riboflavin, chromium, calcium, vitamin D, vitamin C, vitamin B_6, thiamine, folic acid, niacin, and ginger have also been reported to be helpful for migraines, but the scientific evidence is weak to nonexistent.

Other Treatments

Identifying and eliminating allergenic foods from your diet appears to be helpful in reducing the frequency of migraine attacks.[26]

At least one small double-blind study using real and "sham" treatment suggests that acupuncture can reduce the intensity and number of migraine attacks.[27] Furthermore, the improvements were found to continue for at least a year after the cessation of acupuncture treatment.

NAUSEA

Principal Natural Treatments
Ginger
Other Natural Treatments
Vitamin C, vitamin K, lowfat diet

Nausea can be caused by many factors, including stomach flu, viral infections of the inner ear (labyrinthitis), motion sickness, pregnancy, and chemotherapy. If you are continually nauseous, it can be more disabling than chronic pain. Successful treatment can make an enormous difference in your quality of life.

The sensation of nausea can originate in either the nervous system or the digestive tract itself. Most conventional treatments for nausea, such as Dramamine and Compazine, act on the nervous system, but products like Pepto-Bismol soothe the digestive tract directly.

Principal Natural Treatments for Nausea
The herb ginger has become a widely accepted treatment for nausea.

Ginger: May Help Several Types of Nausea

Native to southern Asia, ginger is a 2- to 4-foot perennial that produces grass-like leaves up to a foot long and almost an inch wide. Ginger root, as it is named in the grocery store, actually consists of the underground stem of the plant with its bark-like outer covering scraped off.

Ginger has been used as food and medicine for millennia. Ginger's modern use dates back to the early 1980s, when a scientist named D. Mowrey noticed that ginger-filled capsules reduced his nausea during an episode of flu. Subsequent research ultimately led Germany's Commission E to approve ginger as a treatment for indigestion and motion sickness.

Ginger is typically not as effective as standard drugs for motion sickness, but it has the advantage of not causing drowsiness. Some physicians recommend ginger over other motion sickness drugs for older individuals who are unusually sensitive to drowsiness or loss of balance.

Ginger is also used for the nausea and vomiting of pregnancy, and some conventional medical textbooks mention it. However, physicians are hesitant to recommend any treatment during pregnancy until full safety studies have been performed, and although it is a food, these studies have not yet been completed for ginger (see the following discussion).

European physicians sometimes give their patients ginger before and just after surgery to prevent the nausea that many people experience when they awaken from anesthesia. However, this treatment should be attempted only with a physician's approval.

What Is the Scientific Evidence for Ginger?

Scientific evidence suggests that ginger can be helpful for various forms of nausea.

Nausea and Vomiting of Pregnancy A preliminary double-blind study performed in Denmark concluded that ginger can significantly reduce the nausea and vomiting that often accompany pregnancy.[1] Effects became apparent in 19 of 27 women after 4 days of treatment.

Motion Sickness The first scientific study of ginger for motion sickness followed 36 college students with a known tendency toward motion sickness.[2] They were treated with either ginger or the standard antinausea drug dimenhydrinate and then placed in a rotating chair to see how much motion they could stand. Both treatments seemed about equally effective. Another study also found equivalent benefit between ginger and dimenhydrinate in a group of 60 passengers on a cruise through rough seas.[3] A study of 79 Swedish naval cadets found that ginger could decrease vomiting and cold sweating, but it didn't significantly decrease nausea and vertigo.[4]

However, a 1984 study funded by NASA found that ginger was not any more effective than placebo at reducing the symptoms of nausea caused by a vigorous nausea-provoking method.[5] Negative results were also seen in another study that used a strong nausea stimulus.[6]

Put all together, these studies paint a picture of a treatment that is somewhat effective for motion sickness, but cannot overcome severe nausea.

Post-Surgical Nausea A double-blind British study compared the effects of ginger, placebo, and the drug metoclopramide in the treatment of nausea following gynecological surgery.[7] The results in 60 women showed that both treatments produced similar benefits compared to placebo.

A similar British study followed 120 women receiving gynecological surgery.[8] Whereas nausea and vomiting developed in 41% of participants given a placebo, in the groups treated with ginger or metoclopramide (Reglan), these symptoms developed in only 21% and 27%, respectively.

However, a double-blind study of 108 people undergoing similar surgery showed no benefit with ginger as compared to placebo.[9] Negative results were also seen in another study.[10]

Warning: Do not use ginger either before or immediately after surgery or labor and delivery without a physician's approval. Not only is it important to have an empty stomach before undergoing anesthesia, there are theoretical concerns that ginger may affect bleeding.

Dosage

For most purposes, the standard dosage of powdered ginger is 1 to 4 g daily taken in 2 to 4 divided doses.

To prevent motion sickness, it is probably best to begin treatment 1 or 2 days before the trip and continue it throughout the period of travel.

In the nausea and vomiting of pregnancy, the best form of ginger is probably freshly brewed tea made from boiled ginger root or powdered ginger and diluted to taste. If chilled, carbonated, and sweetened, this would become the original form of ginger ale, a famous antinausea beverage.

Safety Issues

Ginger is on the FDA's "generally recognized as safe" (GRAS) list and seldom causes any side effects.

Like onions and garlic, extracts of ginger interfere with blood clotting in test tubes. This has led to a theoretical concern that ginger should not be combined with drugs such as Coumadin (warfarin), Trental (pentoxifylline), or even aspirin. However, European studies with actual oral ginger in normal quantities have not found any effect on clotting.[11,12,13]

Maximum safe dosages for young children, pregnant or nursing women, or those with severe liver or kidney disease have not been established.

Other Natural Treatments for Nausea

Although the following natural treatments are widely recommended to relieve nausea, there is as yet little scientific evidence that they work.

Vitamin K and Vitamin C

On the basis of studies conducted in the 1950s, a combination of vitamin K (5 mg) and vitamin C (25 mg) is sometimes recommended for morning sickness.[14] Please keep in mind that supplemental vitamin K can interfere with prescription blood-thinning drugs, such as Coumadin (warfarin) and heparin.

Other Recommendations

Diets high in saturated fat (animal fat) can increase morning sickness in some people.[15]

NIGHT VISION
(Impaired)

Principal Natural Treatments
Bilberry
Other Natural Treatments
Grape seed PCOs, vitamin A, zinc

The ability to see in poor light depends on the presence of a substance in the eye called rhodopsin, or visual purple. It is destroyed by bright light but rapidly regenerates in the dark. However, for some people, the adaptation to darkness or the recovery from glare takes an unusually long time. There is no medical treatment for this condition.

Principal Natural Treatments for Impaired Night Vision

The herb bilberry is widely used as a treatment for impaired night vision. However, the scientific evidence is not yet as strong as it should be.

Bilberry: Widely Used in Europe for Impaired Night Vision

The herb bilberry, a close relative of the American blueberry, is the most commonly mentioned natural treatment for impaired night vision. This use dates back to World War II, when pilots in Britain's Royal Air Force reported that a good dose of bilberry jam just before a mission improved their night vision, often dramatically. After the war, medical researchers investigated the constituents of bilberry and found some evidence that it might be effective.

Two preliminary placebo-controlled studies of bilberry found that the herb improved vision in semidarkness, shortened time necessary to adapt to darkness, and speeded recovery from glare.[1,2] Other studies that did not have a placebo group have also found benefits.[3,4,5]

The effects of bilberry are believed to be due to a group of chemicals called anthocyanosides. These naturally occurring antioxidants have a special attraction to the retina.[6]

The standard dosage of bilberry is 160 mg twice daily of an extract standardized to contain 25% bilberry anthocyanosides.

As one might expect of a food, bilberry is quite safe. Enormous quantities have been administered to rats without toxic effects.[7,8] One study involving 2,295 participants showed no serious side effects and only a 4% occurrence of mild reactions, such as gastrointestinal distress, skin rashes, and drowsiness.[9] However, safety in young children, pregnant or nursing women, and those with severe liver or kidney disease has not been established.

Bilberry has no known drug interactions. However, bilberry anthocyanosides, like other common flavonoids, mildly interfere with blood clotting. For this reason, high doses of concentrated bilberry extract might not be appropriate for individuals taking strong blood-thinning drugs, such as Coumadin (warfarin) and heparin.

Other Natural Treatments for Impaired Night Vision

Extracts of grape seed have also been recommended for improving night vision. (See the discussion under Varicose Veins for more information on grape seed.)

There is no question that deficiencies of vitamin A and zinc can also negatively affect night vision. Since zinc is commonly lacking in many people's diets, taking 15 to 20 mg of zinc daily (along with 1 to 3 mg of copper for balance) may be advisable.

OSTEOARTHRITIS

Principal Natural Treatments

Glucosamine, chondroitin sulfate, S-adenosylmethionine

Other Natural Treatments

Devil's claw, healthy diet, boswellia, turmeric, yucca, white willow, boron, vitamin B_6, vitamin D, niacinamide, pantothenic acid, copper, D-phenylalanine, selenium, molybdenum, zinc

In osteoarthritis (OA), the cartilage in joints has become damaged, disrupting the smooth gliding motion of the joint surfaces. The result is pain, swelling, and deformity.

The pain of OA typically increases with joint use and improves at rest. For reasons that aren't clear, although x rays can find evidence of arthritis, the level of pain and stiffness experienced by people does not match the extent of injury noticed on x rays.

Many theories exist about the causes of OA, but we don't really know what causes the disease. OA is often described as "wear and tear" arthritis. However, evidence suggests that this simple explanation is not correct. For example, OA frequently develops in many joints at the same time, often symmetrically on both sides of the body, even when there is no reason to believe that equal amounts of wear and tear are present. Another intriguing finding is that OA of the knee is commonly (and mysteriously) associated with OA of the hand. These factors, as well as others, have led to the suggestion that OA may actually be a body-wide disease of the cartilage.

During one's lifetime, cartilage is constantly being turned over by a balance of forces that both break down and rebuild it. One prevailing theory suggests that OA may represent a situation in which the degrading forces get out of hand. Some of the proposed natural treatments for OA described later may inhibit enzymes that damage cartilage.

When the cartilage damage in OA begins, the body responds by building new cartilage. For several years, this compensating effort can keep the joint functioning well. Some of the natural treatments described below appear to work by assisting the body in repairing cartilage. Eventually, however, building forces cannot keep up with destructive ones, and what is called end-stage OA develops. This is the familiar picture of pain and impaired joint function.

The conventional medical treatment for OA consists mainly of analgesic medications, such as Tylenol, and anti-inflammatory drugs, such as Aleve and Orudis. The main problem with anti-inflammatory drugs is that they can cause ulcers. Another possible problem is that they may actually speed the progression of osteoarthritis by interfering with cartilage repair and promoting cartilage destruction.[1-5] In contrast, at least two of the treatments described below may actually slow the course of the disease, although this hasn't been conclusively proven.

Recently, the use of extracts of cayenne pepper has found its way into conventional medicine. Briefly, it consists of the regular application of cayenne cream to the affected joint, ultimately resulting in a decreased sensation of pain. Unfortunately, this truly natural treatment seldom provides more than modest relief.

Principal Natural Treatments for Osteoarthritis

There are several very useful natural treatments for osteoarthritis. Not only do they reduce pain without causing any side effects, some may actually slow the progression of OA.

Glucosamine: Safe Pain Relief That Lasts

One of the best-documented alternative approaches to the treatment of OA is the supplement glucosamine. Glucosamine is a small molecule formed of a sugar attached to a chemical structure called an amine. Taking glucosamine supplements provides a natural raw material for rebuilding cartilage. It seems to stimulate the activity of cartilage cells and perhaps also protect cartilage from damage.[6-13]

In Portugal, Spain, and Italy, glucosamine has been a primary treatment for OA since the 1980s, and it is also widely used by veterinarians in the United States. Many European physicians believe that it may actually slow the course of the disease, and for this reason they call it a "chondroprotective" drug ("chondro" refers to cartilage). Unfortunately, this wonderful possibility has not been proven. We have more evidence for chondroitin (see the following section).

What Is the Scientific Evidence for Glucosamine?

Reasonably solid studies have found that supplementation with glucosamine sulfate can relieve the pain of OA. For example, one recent double-blind study compared the effectiveness of glucosamine sulfate and placebo in 252 people with OA of the knee.[14] The results showed that after 4 weeks the participants treated with glucosamine sulfate were in less pain and could move better than those given a placebo. No more side effects were noted in the participants who took glucosamine than in those who did not.

Another study found glucosamine equally effective to the standard arthritis drug Feldene.[15] A total of 329 participants were given 20 mg of Feldene, glucosamine, a placebo, or glucosamine plus Feldene daily. Improvement was monitored through the Lequesne Index, a rating scale that evaluates the severity of OA. Equivalent benefit was seen in all the treated groups. After 90 days, treatment was then stopped, and the participants were followed for an additional 8 weeks.

Interestingly, whereas the benefits of Feldene rapidly disappeared following the end of treatment, glucosamine was still producing a full effect at the end of the post-treatment period.

Other studies, enrolling a total of more than 350 participants, have found equivalent benefit between glucosamine and low doses of ibuprofen.[16,17]

Dosage

Glucosamine is usually taken as glucosamine sulfate, at a dosage of 500 mg 3 times daily. It is not truly a cure because it must be taken forever for good results. It also does not produce complete relief. However, it often appears to help significantly. Pain ordinarily begins to improve in about a week and the benefit continues to increase for a month or more.

Safety Issues

Glucosamine is believed to be nontoxic and essentially side-effect free.[18,19] This gives it a huge potential advantage over standard drug treatment, which can cause ulcers.

Chondroitin Sulfate: Relieves Pain
and May Slow Progression of Osteoarthritis

Reasonably good evidence supports the use of chondroitin sulfate for the pain of osteoarthritis as well. In addition, provocative evidence suggests that it may help prevent your arthritis from gradually getting worse.

Like glucosamine, chondroitin plays a natural role in the body's manufacture of cartilage. In Europe, chondroitin sulfate is usually injected directly into arthritic joints (under no circumstances should you try this yourself!). However, in the United States, oral chondroitin sulfate is the most popular form of this supplement.

For years it was questioned whether oral chondroitin sulfate could possibly work. Because of its large molecular size it is difficult to see how chondroitin sulfate could find its way through the lining of the digestive tract to be absorbed into the bloodstream. However, in 1995 researchers found evidence that up to 15% of chondroitin is actually absorbed.[20]

Scientists are unsure how chondroitin sulfate works, but one of two theories (or both) might explain its mode of action. Some evidence suggests that chondroitin may inhibit the enzymes that break down cartilage in the joints.[21] Another theory holds that chondroitin sulfate increases the amount of hyaluronic acid in the joints. Hyaluronic acid is a protective fluid that keeps the joints lubricated.

Perhaps the most exciting development is the recent evidence suggesting that chondroitin sulfate can actually slow the progression of osteoarthritis. This would make it a true chondroprotective drug (see the discussion under Glucosamine). However, more research is needed.

Chondroitin sulfate is often sold in combination with glucosamine. Unfortunately, we have no direct evidence that taking both supplements at once is better than taking just one or the other.

What Is the Scientific Evidence for Chondroitin Sulfate?

Much of the early research on chondroitin sulfate was published in French or Italian journals, and has not been translated into English. However, the results of four double-blind placebo-controlled clinical trials were recently published in English. They provide substantial evidence that chondroitin sulfate is an effective treatment for osteoarthritis. Some show evidence that chondroitin sulfate can reduce the symptoms of OA, while others suggest that it can actually stop the disease from progressing.

Reducing Symptoms Studies, involving a total of more than 250 people and lasting from 3 months to 1 year, have found chondroitin effective for reducing the symptoms of arthritis.

A recent 6-month double-blind placebo-controlled study followed 85 individuals with osteoarthritis of the knee.[22] Participants received either 400 mg of chondroitin sulfate twice a day or placebo. Researchers evaluated improvement in arthritis symptoms by recording the level of pain as judged by the participant, the need for other medications, the time necessary to walk 20 meters on flat ground, and the overall effectiveness of the treatment as rated by physicians and participants.

After 1 month of treatment there was a 23% decrease in joint pain in the chondroitin sulfate group versus only a 12% decrease in the placebo group. By 6 months there was a 43% improvement in the chondroitin sulfate group versus only a 3% improvement in the placebo group (the placebo effect seems to have worn off after a while). Walking speed remained the same for the chondroitin sulfate group, while in the placebo group walking speed gradually and steadily declined. Finally, physicians judged the improvement as good or very good in 69% of those taking chondroitin sulfate, but only 32% of those taking placebo.

Another study enrolled 127 participants for a period of 3 months and also found positive results.[23] A third double-blind study involved only 42 participants, but followed them for a full year. Chondroitin sulfate took months to reach its full effect, but eventually relieved symptoms considerably better than placebo.[24]

Slowing the Disease An exciting feature of this last study was that individuals taking a placebo showed progressive joint damage over the year, but among those taking chondroitin sulfate no worsening of the joints was seen. In other words, chondroitin sulfate seemed to protect the joints of osteoarthritis sufferers from further damage.

No conventional treatment for osteoarthritis protects joints or slows the progression of the disease. If confirmed by larger, properly designed studies, this effect may make chondroitin sulfate a distinctly superior treatment to NSAIDs (nonsteroidal anti-inflammatory drugs) or other conventional medications.

A longer and larger double-blind placebo-controlled trial also found evidence that chondroitin sulfate can slow the progression of OA.[25] One hundred and nineteen people were enrolled in this study, which lasted a full 3 years. Thirty-four of the participants received 1,200 mg of chondroitin sulfate per day; the rest received placebo. Over the course of the study researchers took x rays to determine how many joints had progressed to a severe stage.

During the 3 years of the study only 8.8% of those who took chondroitin sulfate developed severely damaged joints, whereas almost 30% of those who took placebo progressed to this extent. Unfortunately, the report did not state whether this difference was statistically significant.

Additional evidence comes from animal studies. Researchers measured the effects of chondroitin sulfate (administered both orally and via injection directly into the muscle) in rabbits, in which cartilage damage had been induced in one knee by the injection of an enzyme.[26] After 84 days of treatment, the damaged knees in the animals who had been given chondroitin sulfate had significantly more cartilage left than the knees of the untreated animals. Giving chondroitin sulfate by mouth was as effective as giving it through an injection.

Putting It All Together

Looking at the sum of the evidence, it does appear that chondroitin sulfate may actually protect joints from damage in osteoarthritis. However, better studies are needed to confirm this very important potential benefit. Furthermore, none of this work demonstrates any power to reverse the disease by rebuilding the cartilage. Chondroitin sulfate may simply stop further destruction from occurring, but that in itself is excellent.

Dosage

The usual dosage of chondroitin sulfate is 400 mg taken 3 times daily. It is frequently combined with glucosamine in commercial products, although there is no direct evidence that such combinations are more effective than either treatment alone.

Safety Issues

Chondroitin sulfate has not been associated with any serious adverse effects. Subjects in clinical trials have found mild digestive system distress to be the only real complaint.

S-Adenosylmethionine: Helpful, but Very Expensive

S-adenosylmethionine (SAMe) is a substance that occurs naturally in the body, and plays a role in numerous biochemical functions. When used for osteoarthritis, it appears to reduce pain, decrease swelling, and improve mobility about as effectively as standard anti-inflammatory drugs, with significantly fewer side effects and risks. There is also some evidence that SAMe may slow the progression of osteoarthritis. However, this is an extraordinarily expensive supplement.

What Is the Scientific Evidence for SAMe?

A great deal of good scientific evidence supports the use of S-adenosylmethionine (SAMe) in arthritis.[27] Numerous double-blind studies involving over a thousand participants in total suggest that it is approximately as effective as standard anti-inflammatory drugs.

One of the best double-blind studies enrolled 734 patients and followed them for 4 weeks.[28] Over this period, 235 of the participants received 1,200 mg of SAMe per day, while a similar number took either placebo or 750 mg daily of the standard drug naproxen. The majority of these patients had experienced moderate symptoms of OA of either the knee or of the hip for an average of 6 years.

The results indicate that SAMe provided as much pain-relieving effect as naproxen, and that both treatments were significantly better than the placebo. However, differences did exist between the two treatments. Naproxen worked more quickly, producing readily apparent benefits at the 2-week follow-up, whereas the full effect of SAMe was not apparent until 4 weeks. By the end of the study, both treatments were producing the same level of benefit. We do not know whether further improvement would have been seen in the SAMe group had the study continued longer, or whether the benefits would have faded away.

Animal evidence suggests that SAMe may help protect cartilage from damage.[29,30]

Dosage

SAMe is usually started at an initial dosage of 200 mg twice daily, which is then increased over 1 to 2 weeks up to 1,200 mg per day. The reason for this gradual approach is that if full doses are taken from the beginning many people develop stomach distress.

After symptoms improve, doses as low as 200 mg twice daily may suffice to keep pain under control.

Safety Issues

SAMe appears to be very safe in general, both in the short and long term.[31–35]

However, people with bipolar disease should not use SAMe except under medical supervision.[36,37] The reason is that SAMe also appears to have antidepressant properties, and, like other antidepressants, can cause people with bipolar disease to enter a manic state.

Safety in young children, pregnant or nursing women, or those with severe liver or renal disease has not been fully established. However, SAMe has been studied in pregnant women.[38]

It has been suggested that SAMe might interact with various drugs (technically, by facilitating their conjugation),[39] but this has not been proven to cause any actual problem. SAMe should definitely not be combined with prescription antidepressants except under the supervision of a physician.[40]

Other Natural Treatments for Osteoarthritis

The following natural treatments are widely recommended for osteoarthritis, but they have not yet been scientifically proven effective.

Devil's Claw: Reduces Arthritis Pain

Several preliminary double-blind studies involving a total of over 200 people suggest that the herb devil's claw can soothe the pain of various types of arthritis.[41]

A typical dosage of devil's claw is 750 mg 3 times daily of a preparation standardized to contain 3% iridoid glycosides. Devil's claw appears to be quite safe, with no evidence of toxicity at doses many times higher than recommended.[42] A 6-month open study of 630 people with arthritis who took devil's claw showed no side effects other than occasional mild gastrointestinal distress.[43] For the latter reason, it is recommended that those with ulcers not take devil's claw.

Safety in young children, pregnant or nursing women, or those with severe liver or kidney disease has not been established.

Healthy Diet: Can Slow the Progression of Arthritis

There is considerable evidence that a diet high in vitamins C and E and beta-carotene can slow the progression of osteoarthritis, by as much as 70%.[44] These nutrients are found in fruits, vegetables, whole grains, nuts, and seeds. However, we don't know whether taking supplements is just as effective. As described in detail under Cancer, when you get vitamins from foods you also get numerous other healthful substances.

Miscellaneous Herbs and Supplements

Weak evidence suggests that the herbs boswellia, turmeric, and yucca may be useful for OA. (See *The Natural Pharmacist: Your Complete Guide to Herbs* for more information.)

The herb white willow contains aspirin-like substances and thus might be helpful. However, whether enough of these natural anti-inflammatories are provided by standard doses of white willow to produce adequate pain relief has not been documented. White willow may irritate the stomach lining like aspirin, and for that reason should not be taken by those with stomach ulcers. Other aspirin warnings apply as well: White willow should not be used by people with aspirin allergies, bleeding disorders, kidney disease, liver disease, or diabetes. It may also interact adversely with alcohol, "blood thinners," other anti-inflammatories, methotrexate, metoclopramide, phenytoin, probenecid, spironolactone, and valproate.

Other substances sometimes recommended for OA include boron, vitamin B_6, vitamin D, niacinamide, pantothenic acid, copper, D-phenylalanine, selenium, molybdenum, and zinc.

(For more information on arthritis, see *The Natural Pharmacist Guide to Arthritis.*)

OSTEOPOROSIS

Principal Natural Treatments
Calcium, vitamin D, ipriflavone, trace minerals, essential fatty acids
Other Natural Treatments
Copper, magnesium, strontium, vitamins B_6 and B_{12}, vitamin K, folic acid, boron, progesterone

In centuries past, the fragile bones and stooped stature of the aged were taken for granted. Today, however, prevention of osteoporosis is a real possibility.

Many factors are now known or suspected to accelerate the rate of bone loss. These include smoking, alcohol, low calcium intake, excessive phosphorus intake (such as found in soft drinks), a high-protein diet, lack of exercise, various medications, and several medical illnesses. Women are much more prone to osteoporosis than men and, for this reason, the following discussion focuses almost entirely on them.

Conventional medical treatment for osteoporosis in women centers mainly on hormone-replacement therapy. Although supplemental estrogen undoubtedly slows and perhaps even reverses osteoporosis, recent concern about the increased risk of breast cancer has caused many women and their physicians to rethink the use of this therapy. The so-called designer estrogen raloxifene (Evista) may offer benefits without this risk. Other drugs, such as Fosamax (a nonhormonal drug), can also help build bone.

Weight-bearing exercise is strongly recommended.

Principal Natural Treatments for Osteoporosis

There is good evidence that calcium supplements may be able to slow the progression of osteoporosis. A combination of calcium and vitamin D may be able to produce even better effects, and it appears that the semisynthetic substance ipriflavone can actually reverse the disease to some extent. The combination of ipriflavone and calcium has also been tested and found more effective than calcium alone.

Calcium and Vitamin D

Calcium is necessary to build and maintain bone. You need vitamin D, too, as the body cannot absorb calcium without it. (Although your body can manufacture vitamin D when exposed to the sun, in this age of sunblock, supplemental vitamin D may be necessary.)

Numerous good studies indicate that calcium supplements can help prevent and slow osteoporosis.[1] Calcium supplementation at the recommended doses appears to be able to reduce bone loss in postmenopausal women in every bone site except the spine.[2,3] Good evidence also tells us that when vitamin D is taken along with calcium the results are even better.[4] Combination treatment may be able to slow osteoporosis in the spine, and in some cases actually reverse osteoporosis to some extent.

While estrogen is more powerful than calcium alone, taking calcium along with estrogen offers additional benefits.[5,6] Calcium supplements also help adolescent girls "put calcium in the bank."[7]

Adding various trace minerals (zinc, 15 mg; copper, 2.5 mg; and manganese, 5 mg) along with calcium and vitamin D seems to produce further improvement.[8,9] Essential fatty acids (fish oil and evening primrose oil) may also enhance the effectiveness of calcium.[10,11]

Dosage

Appropriate dietary intake of calcium is as follows: 400 mg daily for infants; 800 mg daily for children up to the age of 19; 1,000 mg daily for adults up to the age 50; and 1,200 mg of calcium per day for adults over 50, as well as pregnant or nursing women. Because calcium competes with the absorption of other minerals, you should consider taking a multimineral supplement as well.

The usual recommendation for vitamin D is 400 IU daily. However, some of the studies cited here used dosages as high as 800 IU daily. Such doses should be taken only with medical supervision.

Safety Issues

In general, a daily intake of calcium up to 2,000 mg is safe.[12] However, if you have cancer, hyperparathyroidism, or sarcoidosis, you should only take calcium under the supervision of a physician.

Those with kidney stones or a history of kidney stones are often cautioned not to take supplemental calcium. The reason for this warning is that kidney stones are commonly made of calcium oxalate crystals. Recent studies, however, have found no relationship between increased calcium intake and the occurrence of kidney stones.[13] In fact, some studies show that kidney stone risk actually goes down with the use of calcium.[14]

Vitamin D is safe when taken at a dosage of 400 IU daily, but can be toxic when taken at doses higher than 1,000 IU daily. Individuals with sarcoidosis or hyperparathyroidism should not take vitamin D except on medical advice.

Ipriflavone

Various plants contain estrogen-like substances known as phytoestrogens. In 1969, a research project was started to manufacture a type of phytoestrogen that would cause the bone-stimulating effects of phytoestrogens but not the other effects of estrogen. The purpose behind this search was to find a treatment that could prevent osteoporosis without incurring any of estrogen's risks.

The starting point was the research of the phytoestrogens found in soy, called isoflavones. Scientists eventually developed a semisynthetic variation of soy isoflavones named ipriflavone. After 7 successful years of animal experiments with ipriflavone, human research was started in 1981. Today, ipriflavone is available in over 22 countries. Drugstores in the United States can now carry it as a nonprescription dietary supplement.

Ipriflavone appears to help prevent osteoporosis by interfering with the growth of osteoclasts, cells that cause bone breakdown. Estrogen works in much the same way. But, as was intended by its inventors, ipriflavone does not appear to produce estrogenic effects anywhere else in the body. For this reason, it probably doesn't increase the risk of breast or uterine cancer. However, it also doesn't reduce hot flashes, night sweats, mood changes, or vaginal dryness.

What Is the Scientific Evidence for Ipriflavone?

Numerous double-blind placebo-controlled studies involving a total of over 1,000 participants have examined the effects of ipriflavone on osteoporosis.[15–20] Overall, it appears that ipriflavone can stop the progression of osteoporosis and perhaps reverse it to some extent.

For example, a 2-year double-blind study followed 198 postmenopausal women who had evidence of bone loss.[21] At the end of the study, there was a gain in bone density of

1% in the ipriflavone group compared to a loss of 0.7% in the placebo group.

Taking calcium plus ipriflavone may also be an excellent idea. In one study, 60 women, who had already been diagnosed with osteoporosis and had already suffered one spinal fracture, were given either 1,000 mg of calcium or 1,000 mg of calcium with ipriflavone.[22] After 6 months, the ipriflavone group had an increase of bone density in the spine of 3.5%, compared to a 2.1% net loss in the calcium-only group.

Ipriflavone may also be helpful for preventing osteoporosis in women who are taking Lupron, a medication that accelerates bone loss.[23]

Finally, there is some evidence that combining ipriflavone with estrogen may improve anti-osteoporosis benefits.[24,25] However, we do not know whether such combinations enhance or diminish estrogen's other benefits, such as reducing heart disease.

Dosage

The proper dosage of ipriflavone has been well established through studies: 200 mg 3 times daily or 300 mg 2 times daily. (A lower dose is necessary for those with kidney failure. Please consult your physician for details.)

Safety Issues

To date, 2,769 people have been treated with ipriflavone, for an average duration of more than one year. The incidence of side effects in those treated with ipriflavone was no more than what was observed in those taking placebo.[26]

However, because ipriflavone is eliminated by the kidneys, concerns have been raised about the use of ipriflavone by patients with kidney problems.

Ipriflavone does not appear to affect the uterus, brain, breast, or vaginal tissue of postmenopausal women or the thyroid gland and uterus of experimental animals.[27]

However, given the lack of large long-term cancer-risk studies for ipriflavone, women who have had breast cancer should use ipriflavone only on a physician's advice.

Other Natural Treatments for Osteoporosis

A wide variety of other food supplements have also been suggested as useful for the prevention or reversal of osteoporosis, including copper; magnesium; strontium; vitamins B_6, B_{12}, and K; and folic acid. However, the evidence for the effectiveness of these methods is quite weak.

Boron is frequently mentioned as a treatment for osteoporosis as well. However, there are some concerns that boron may raise estrogen levels, and therefore might present an increased risk of cancer. [28,29]

The Progesterone Story

Many books promote the idea that natural progesterone prevents or even reduces osteoporosis. (In this case, the term *natural* indicates that we are using the same progesterone found in the body. The "progesterone" found in conventional medications consists not of progesterone itself, but of its chemical cousins known as progestins. These are used because they are much more absorbable orally than true progesterone. But when you purchase true progesterone, it too is made synthetically.)

However, although theoretical evidence does suggest that progesterone may help build bone,[30] no properly performed studies have been done to test whether supplementation with progesterone actually helps osteoporosis.

PERIODONTAL DISEASE
(Gum Disease)

Principal Natural Treatments

Coenzyme Q_{10}

Other Natural Treatments

Folic acid mouthwash, zinc, vitamin C, calcium, magnesium, vitamin B_{12}

Periodontal disease begins with gum inflammation and progresses to pockets of infection, bone loss, and loosening of the teeth. It is present in 90% of individuals over the age of 65.

Conventional prevention and treatment include regular flossing, using mouthwash that contains extracts of the herb thyme (such as thymol, found in Listerine), and using special toothbrushing appliances. If the condition becomes advanced, special deep-cleaning techniques and even surgery may be necessary.

Principal Natural Treatments for Periodontal Disease

The supplement coenzyme Q_{10} (CoQ_{10}), more widely known as a treatment for heart-related conditions, is also used for periodontal disease.

Coenzyme Q_{10}

Several preliminary studies suggest that the supplement coenzyme Q_{10} can help periodontal disease.[1–6]

For example, in one double-blind study, 56 individuals received either 60 mg CoQ_{10} or placebo for 4 weeks. The results showed that coenzyme Q10 significantly improved signs of periodontal disease, specifically the depth of gum "pockets."[7] The proper dosage of CoQ_{10} is 50 to 100 mg daily. CoQ_{10} is essentially side-effect free. (For more information, see the discussion under Congestive Heart Failure.)

Other Natural Treatments for Periodontal Disease

The following natural treatments are widely recommended for periodontal disease, but they have not been scientifically proven effective at this time.

Folic Acid

Preliminary studies suggest that folic acid mouthwash may help in periodontal disease as well. Oral folic acid supplementation does not appear to be especially effective.[8–11]

Other Supplements

Other common recommendations include zinc, vitamin C, calcium, magnesium, and vitamin B_{12}. However, none of these suggestions has any significant research basis.

PMS
(Premenstrual Stress Syndrome)

Principal Natural Treatments
Calcium, chasteberry

Other Natural Treatments
Vitamin E, magnesium, multivitamin and mineral supplements, evening primrose oil (for cyclic breast tenderness), ginkgo, progesterone cream

Probably Ineffective Treatments
Vitamin B_6

Many women experience a variety of unpleasant symptoms in the week or two before menstruating. These include irritability, anger, headaches, anxiety, depression, fatigue, fluid retention, and breast tenderness. These symptoms undoubtedly result from hormonal changes of the menstrual cycle, but we don't know the cause of PMS or exactly how to treat it.

Conventional treatments include antidepressants, antianxiety drugs, beta-blockers, diuretics, oral contraceptives, and other hormonally active formulations. None of these treatments is entirely effective, except for those that take the drastic step of inducing artificial menopause.

Principal Natural Treatments for PMS

There is fairly good evidence that calcium supplements can significantly reduce all the major symptoms of PMS. There is also some evidence that the herbs chasteberry and ginkgo can lessen the symptoms of PMS. Vitamin B_6 is widely recommended as well, but its scientific record is mixed at best. (For more detailed information on PMS, see *The Natural Pharmacist Guide to PMS*.)

Calcium: May Improve All Symptoms of PMS

A recent study found surprisingly positive results using calcium (1,200 mg daily) for the treatment of PMS symptoms. These results have made a big impact because the study was large (500 women) and was performed at a prestigious medical center, Columbia University.[1]

Participants took 300 mg of calcium (as calcium carbonate) 4 times daily. Compared to placebo, calcium significantly reduced mood swings, pain, bloating, depression, back pain, and food cravings. Similar findings were also seen in earlier preliminary studies.[2,3]

For healthy women, calcium is safe when taken at this dosage. However, if you have cancer, hyperparathyroidism, or sarcoidosis, you should only take calcium under the supervision of a physician.

Chasteberry: Especially Effective for Breast Tenderness

The herb chasteberry is widely used in Europe as a treatment for PMS symptoms. More than most herbs, chasteberry is frequently called by its Latin names: *vitex* or *Vitex agnus-castus*. A shrub in the verbena family, chasteberry is commonly found on riverbanks and nearby foothills in central Asia and around the Mediterranean Sea. After its violet flowers have bloomed, a dark brown, peppercorn-size fruit develops, with a pleasant odor reminiscent of peppermint. It is the fruit that is used medicinally.

The modern use of chasteberry dates back to the 1950s, when the German pharmaceutical firm Madaus Company first produced a standardized extract. It has become a standard European treatment for PMS, cyclical breast tenderness, and menstrual irregularities.

Reportedly, chasteberry can reduce many of the symptoms of PMS, but it is probably most dramatically effective for breast tenderness. This is probably because chasteberry suppresses the release of prolactin, a hormone that affects the breasts. Unlike other herbs used for women's health problems, research has shown that chasteberry does not contain any chemicals that act like estrogen or progesterone. Rather, it acts on the pituitary gland to suppress the release of prolactin.[4–7] Prolactin naturally rises during pregnancy to stimulate milk production and other physiological changes.

What Is the Scientific Evidence for Chasteberry?

Chasteberry is widely used in Germany as a general treatment for PMS. However, the scientific record for chasteberry lacks properly designed double-blind studies.

German gynecologists clearly believe that chasteberry is effective for PMS. In surveys involving about 3,000 women who had been prescribed chasteberry, physicians rated the overall effect of the treatment as good or very good 92% of the time.[8,9] Based on the women's own reports, good results were seen in 57% of participants, but only 33% reported complete relief. Chasteberry appears to be particularly effective in reducing the cyclic breast pain of PMS.[10]

However, these were not double-blind studies. Since there is a very high level of placebo response in PMS, often reaching 70%,[11] proper double-blind studies are necessary to determine the actual effectiveness of chasteberry.

A recently reported double-blind study followed 175 women with PMS for 3 months. Half of them received a standard chasteberry preparation, and the other half took 200 mg of pyridoxine (vitamin B_6) daily.[12] Over the 3-month study period, chasteberry was associated with "a considerably more marked alleviation of typical PMS complaints, such as breast tenderness, edema, inner tension, headache, constipation and depression." Overall, 77% of the participants treated with chasteberry showed improvement.

However, the level of improvement was rated excellent in only 24.5% of cases; this seems to indicate a relatively low level of effectiveness. Furthermore, pyridoxine may not be an effective treatment for PMS; so the fact that chasteberry proved superior is less significant than it might at first appear (see the discussion under Vitamin B_6).

Dosage

Because there are so many different preparations, chasteberry extract should be taken according to the directions on the label. The herb's full benefits may take months to develop, so be patient.

Safety Issues

No detailed studies of the safety of chasteberry have been conducted. However, its widespread use in Germany has not led to any reports of significant adverse effects,[13] with the exception of a single case of excessive ovarian stimulation possibly caused by chasteberry.[14] In a study of over 1,500 women, mild side effects such as nausea, headache and allergic skin reactions were reported by less than 2.5% of participants.[15]

Because it lowers prolactin levels, chasteberry is not an appropriate treatment for pregnant or nursing mothers. Its safety in adolescents or those with severe liver or kidney disease has not been established.

No known drug interactions are associated with chasteberry. However, it's quite conceivable that the herb could interfere with other hormonal medications, such as birth control pills, or drugs that affect the pituitary, such as bromocriptine.

Vitamin B_6 : May Not Be Effective

Vitamin B_6 has been used for PMS for many decades, both by European and U.S. physicians. However, the results of scientific studies are mixed at best. A recent study found vitamin B_6 ineffective.[16] A dozen or more other double-blind studies have investigated the effectiveness of vitamin B_6 for PMS, but according to a detailed review, overall the negative studies cancel out the positive ones, and all of them suffer from significant scientific flaws.[17] Some books on natural medicine report that the negative studies used too little B_6, but in reality there was no clear link between dosage and effectiveness.

The maximum safe dosage of vitamin B_6 for self-use is 50 mg twice daily. Higher doses should be used only under a physician's supervision because of the potential risk of nerve injury. Some nutritionally oriented physicians

report that the combination of B_6 and magnesium is considerably more effective than either treatment alone (see
the following discussion under Magnesium).

Other Natural Treatments for PMS

The following treatments are widely recommended for
PMS, but they have not yet been scientifically proven
effective.

Vitamin E

Weak evidence suggests that vitamin E may be helpful for
PMS.[18] A typical dosage of vitamin E is 400 IU daily.

Magnesium

Preliminary studies suggest that magnesium may also be
helpful in PMS.[19,20]

Magnesium is usually supplemented in the range of
250 to 500 mg daily, but for PMS it is sometimes given at
a dosage of 1,000 mg daily starting on the day 15 of the
menstrual cycle and continuing through the beginning of
menstruation. This dosage should be safe in healthy
women, but if you suffer from any medical problems, you
should check with a physician before trying it. As mentioned earlier, some physicians believe that magnesium
should be combined with vitamin B_6 for best results.

Multivitamin and Mineral Supplements

Preliminary evidence suggests that combined treatment
with a multivitamin and mineral supplement may be helpful in PMS.[21–24]

Evening Primrose Oil:
Primarily for Cyclic Breast Tenderness

Evening primrose oil is used mainly for the cyclic breast
pain that often occurs with premenstrual syndrome (see

the discussion under Cyclic Mastalgia). It may be helpful with other PMS symptoms as well, but the scientific evidence is weak.[25]

A typical dosage of evening primrose oil is 2 to 3 g daily. It must be taken for at least 4 to 6 weeks for noticeable effect, and maximum benefits may require 4 to 8 months to develop. Evening primrose oil appears to be safe. (For more information about evening primrose oil, see the discussion under Diabetes.)

Ginkgo: For Breast Tenderness and Perhaps Other Symptoms

A recent study suggests that the herb ginkgo can reduce breast tenderness and other symptoms of PMS. (For more information, see Cyclic Mastalgia.)

Additional Treatments

Progesterone cream is another method widely recommended for PMS, but there is little evidence that it is effective.[26]

PSORIASIS

Principal Natural Treatments

There are no well-established natural treatments for psoriasis.

Other Natural Treatments

Fish oil, chromium, selenium, vitamin E, zinc, flaxseed oil, burdock, red clover, *Coleus forskohlii*, goldenseal, milk thistle, fumaric acid, vitamin D, vitamin A

Up to 2% of Americans suffer from psoriasis, a skin condition that leads to an intensely itchy rash with clearly defined borders and scales that resemble silvery mica. The fingernails are also frequently involved, showing pitting or thickening.

Medical treatment for psoriasis includes applications of topical steroids and peeling agents that expose the underlying skin for the steroid to contact. Ultraviolet light can also be used, sometimes combined with coal tar applications or medications called psoralens. Synthetic versions of vitamin A can also be helpful. For especially problematic psoriasis, low doses of the anticancer drug methotrexate have proven quite effective.

Natural Treatments for Psoriasis

The following natural treatments are widely recommended for psoriasis, but they have not been scientifically proven effective at this time.

Fish Oil

There is some evidence that eicosapentaenoic acid (EPA) from fish oil may be a bit helpful in psoriasis. One double-blind study followed 28 people with chronic psoriasis for 8 weeks.[1] Half received 1.8 mg of EPA daily (supplied by 10 capsules of fish oil), and the other half received placebo. By the end of the study, researchers saw significant improvement in itching, redness, and scaling, but not in the size of the psoriasis patches.

Another double-blind study followed 145 people with moderate to severe psoriasis for 4 months.[2] Half received 6 g daily of fish oil supplying 5 g of EPA and docosahexaenoic acid (DHA), and the other half received corn oil as a placebo. After 4 months, neither the participants nor the physicians noticed any improvement in the fish oil group. However, close examination under a microscope showed improvement in scaling and cellular changes in both the fish oil and the corn oil groups.

Fish oil appears to be safe and causes few side effects, except for occasional digestive distress and fishy burps.

However, people with diabetes should use high doses of fish oil only under the supervision of a physician.

Other Herbs and Supplements

Chromium, selenium, vitamin E, zinc, flaxseed oil, burdock, red clover, *Coleus forskohlii,* goldenseal, and milk thistle are mentioned as possible treatments for psoriasis. However, there is no real evidence that they work.

A somewhat toxic natural substance called fumaric acid is sometimes recommended for psoriasis as well. Vitamin D or A taken at high levels may improve symptoms, but these are dangerous treatments that should be used only under the supervision of a physician.

RAYNAUD'S DISEASE

Principal Natural Treatments
There are no well-established natural treatments for Raynaud's disease.
Other Natural Treatments
Inositol hexaniacinate, essential fatty acids, ginkgo

Raynaud's disease is a little understood condition in which the fingers and toes show an exaggerated sensitivity to cold. Classic cases show a characteristic white, blue, and red color sequence as the digits lose blood supply and then rewarm. Some people develop only one or two of these signs.

The cause of Raynaud's disease is unknown. The same symptoms may occur in association with a variety of other diseases, in which case the term *Raynaud's phenomenon* is used instead.

Conventional treatment consists mainly of reassurance and the recommendation to avoid exposure to cold and the use of tobacco (which can worsen Raynaud's). In severe cases, a variety of drugs can be tried.

Natural Treatments for Raynaud's Disease

The following natural treatments are widely recommended for Raynaud's disease, but they have not yet been scientifically proven effective.

Inositol Hexaniacinate

According to one preliminary double-blind study, the special form of niacin called inositol hexaniacinate may be helpful for Raynaud's disease.[1] The dosage used in the study was 4 g daily. At this level of supplementation, regular blood tests to rule out liver inflammation are highly recommended. All forms of niacin may cause facial flushing and affect blood sugar levels in people with diabetes.

Essential Fatty Acids

High doses of fish oil have also shown good results for Raynaud's disease in preliminary double-blind studies.[2,3] However, a very high dosage must be used, perhaps 12 g daily. Do not use cod liver oil, as it will supply too high a dose of vitamins A and D. People with diabetes should not take high doses of fish oil except under medical supervision.

Another preliminary double-blind study suggests that high doses of evening primrose oil may be useful as well.[4,5] (For more information on evening primrose oil use and safety issues, see the discussion under Diabetes.)

When taking essential fatty acids, it is a good idea to take vitamin E as well to prevent the fats from being damaged by free radicals. However, physician supervision is necessary if taking vitamin E in doses higher than 600 IU. (For more information on safety issues concerning vitamin E, see the discussion under Atherosclerosis.)

Ginkgo

Although no direct evidence shows that ginkgo is helpful for Raynaud's disease, it has been shown to increase circulation in the fingertips[6] and thus may be useful. (For more information on ginkgo use and safety issues, see the discussion under Alzheimer's Disease.)

RHEUMATOID ARTHRITIS

Principal Natural Treatments
Fish oil

Other Natural Treatments
Boswellia, devil's claw, curcumin, yucca, GLA, selenium, zinc, boron, magnesium, molybdenum, vitamin C, pantothenic acid, copper, phenylalanine, sea cucumber, cartilage extracts, L-histidine, beta-carotene, ginger, burdock, horsetail, Chinese herbs, dietary changes

---

Rheumatoid arthritis (RA) is an autoimmune disease in the general family of lupus. For reasons that are not understood, in RA the immune system goes awry and begins attacking innocent tissues, especially cartilage in the joints. Various joints become red, hot, and swollen under the onslaught. The pattern of inflammation is usually symmetrical, occurring on both sides of the body. Other symptoms include inflammation of the eyes, nodules or lumps under the skin, and a general feeling of malaise.

RA is more common in women than in men and typically begins between the ages of 35 and 60. The diagnosis is made by matching the pattern of symptoms with certain characteristic laboratory results.

Medical treatment consists mainly of two categories of drugs: anti-inflammatory drugs in the ibuprofen family (nonsteroidal anti-inflammatory drugs, or NSAIDs); and drugs that may be able to put RA into full or partial remission, the so-called disease-modifying antirheumatic drugs (DMARDs).

Anti-inflammatory drugs relieve symptoms of RA but do not change the overall progression of the disease, whereas the DMARDs seem to affect the disease itself. A good analogy might be the various options available to "treat" a house "suffering" from a severe termite infestation. You could remove heavy furniture, tiptoe about instead of holding public dances, and put large beams under the joists. However, none of these methods would do anything to stop the gradual destruction of your house. These methods are like NSAIDs and other supportive techniques in that they treat only the symptoms.

A more definitive approach would be to hire an exterminator and kill the termites. In medical terms, this would be described as a disease-modifying treatment. Because medical treatments for chronic diseases are seldom as completely effective as this example, a closer analogy might be spraying a chemical that slows the spread of termites but does not stop them.

In RA, the drugs believed to alter the course of the disease (to slow it down or stop it) include gold compounds, D-penicillamine, antimalarials, sulfasalazine, and methotrexate. They are unrelated to one another but work somewhat similarly in practice.

Unfortunately, all the drugs in this category are quite toxic and reliably cause severe side effects. Because of this toxicity, for years a so-called pyramid approach was taken with people with RA. Physicians started with NSAIDs to help with the pain and inflammation, and progressed to successively stronger and more toxic medications only when the basic treatments failed. Natural treatments such as those described here might also be useful in early stages.

However, over the last few years, research has found that severe joint damage occurs very early in RA. This evidence has caused many authorities to suggest early, aggressive treatment with disease-modifying drugs to prevent joint damage. Nonetheless, this approach has not been universally adopted, and many physicians still prescribe NSAIDs for early stages of RA. The treatments described here may be reasonable alternative options.

Principal Natural Treatments for Rheumatoid Arthritis

Rheumatoid arthritis is a difficult disease, and no alternative approach solves it easily. Even if you choose to use alternative methods, you should maintain regular visits to a rheumatologist to watch for serious complications. Finally, keep in mind that medical treatment may be able to slow the progression of RA. It is not likely that any of the alternative options have the same power.

Fish Oil

Fish oil is the only natural treatment for RA with significant documentation. According to the results of 12 double-blind placebo-controlled studies involving a total of over 500 participants, supplementation with omega-3 fatty acids can significantly reduce the symptoms of RA.[1]

The most important omega-3 fatty acids found in fish oil are called EPA (eicosapentaenoic acid) and DHA (docosahexaenoic acid). Many forms of fish oil contain about 18% EPA and 12% DHA, for a total of about 30% by weight of omega-3 oils. In order to match the dosage used in several major studies, you should probably take enough fish oil to supply about 1.8 g of EPA (1,800 mg) and 0.9 g (900 mg) of DHA daily. Results may take 3 to 4 months to develop.

There are many forms of fish oil. If you decide to use cod liver oil as your fish oil supplement, make sure you do not exceed the safe maximum intake of vitamins A and D.

These vitamins are fat-soluble, which means that excess amounts tend to build up in your body, potentially reaching toxic levels. The maximum safe daily dosage for vitamin A is 25,000 IU. However, pregnant women should not take more than 10,000 IU of vitamin A daily because of the risk of birth defects. Vitamin D becomes toxic when taken at dosages above 1,000 IU daily for prolonged periods.

Otherwise, fish oil appears to be safe. The most common problem is fishy burps. It does have a mild "blood-thinning" effect, so it should not be combined with strong blood-thinning drugs such as Coumadin (warfarin) and heparin unless so instructed by a physician. However, contrary to some reports, fish oil does not seem to cause bleeding problems when it is taken by itself.[2,3] It also does not appear to raise blood sugar levels in people with diabetes. However, if you have diabetes, you should not take any supplement except on the advice of a physician. Fish oil may temporarily raise the level of LDL ("bad") cholesterol, but this effect seems to be short-lived, and levels return to normal with continued use.[4,5] Flaxseed oil has been offered as a more palatable substitute for fish oil, but there is no evidence that it is effective.

Eating a lot of fish may also be helpful.[6]

Other Natural Treatments for Rheumatoid Arthritis

The following natural treatments are widely recommended for rheumatoid arthritis, but they have not yet been scientifically proven effective.

Boswellia

Boswellia serrata is a shrub-like tree that grows in the dry hills of the Indian subcontinent. It is the source of a resin called salai guggal, which has been used for thousands of years in Ayurvedic medicine, the traditional medicine of the region. It is very similar to a resin from a related tree, *Boswellia carteri*, which is also known as frankincense. Both substances have been used historically for arthritis.

Recent research has identified boswellic acids as the likely active ingredients in boswellia. In animal studies, boswellic acids have shown anti-inflammatory effects, but their mechanism of action seems to be quite different from that of standard anti-inflammatory medications.[7,8]

A recent issue of *Phytomedicine* was devoted to boswellia and briefly reviewed previously unpublished studies on the herb.[9] A pair of placebo-controlled trials involving a total of 81 people with RA found significant reductions in swelling and pain over the course of 3 months. Furthermore, a comparative study of 60 participants over 6 months found the boswellia extract to relieve symptoms about as well as oral gold therapy.

However, the many details of these studies were not described in this summary review. In particular, while gold shots can induce remission in RA, we have no evidence that boswellia can do the same.

Furthermore, another recent double-blind study found no difference between boswellia and placebo.[10] The bottom line is that that we need more research to know for sure whether boswellia is an effective treatment for RA.

The dosage of boswellia most often recommended is 400 mg 3 times a day of an extract that has been standardized to contain 37.5% boswellic acids. The full effect may take as long as 4 to 8 weeks to develop.

Few side effects have been reported with boswellia, other than an occasional allergic reaction or a mild upset stomach. However, due to the lack of formal safety studies, boswellia is not recommended for young children, pregnant or nursing women, or those with severe liver or kidney disease.

Devil's Claw

The herb devil's claw may be beneficial in RA. One double-blind study followed 89 people with RA for 2 months. The group given devil's claw showed a significant decrease in pain intensity and an improvement in mobility.[11]

Another double-blind study of 50 people with various types of arthritis showed that 10 days of treatment with devil's claw provided significant pain relief.[12]

A typical dosage of devil's claw is 750 mg 3 times daily of a preparation standardized to contain 3% iridoid glycosides.

Devil's claw appears to be quite safe, with no evidence of toxicity at doses many times higher than recommended.[13] A 6-month open study of 630 people with arthritis showed no side effects other than occasional mild gastrointestinal distress.[14] However, devil's claw is not advised for those with ulcers. Safety in young children, pregnant or nursing women, and individuals with severe liver or kidney disease has not been established.

Curcumin

Curcumin (an extract of the kitchen spice turmeric) is often suggested as a treatment for RA. Curcumin appears to possess anti-inflammatory properties,[15] and preliminary studies suggest curcumin may relieve symptoms of rheumatoid arthritis,[16] although much more research is needed.

The typical dosage of curcumin is 500 mg 3 times daily. Curcumin is sometimes given in combination with an equal dose of an extract of the pineapple plant called bromelain, which appears to possess anti-inflammatory properties of its own.[17]

Curcumin is thought to be quite safe.[18] Side effects are rare and are generally limited to occasional allergic reactions and mild stomach upset. However, safety in very young children, pregnant or nursing women, and those with severe liver or kidney disease has not been established.

Additional Natural Treatments

One preliminary and rather unimpressive double-blind study suggests that the herb yucca can help relieve the pain of RA.[19]

The essential fatty acid gamma-linolenic acid (GLA), found in evening primrose oil and borage oil, may help relieve symptoms of rheumatoid arthritis.[20] However, to get a high enough dose to be effective, you would probably need to use purified GLA rather than evening primrose oil, and it is not widely available at this time. Selenium has been found helpful in some studies,[21] but not in others.[22,23] The same may be said of zinc.[24,25,26]

The following treatments are also sometimes proposed as effective for rheumatoid arthritis, but there is essentially no scientific evidence to turn to: boron, magnesium, molybdenum, vitamin C, pantothenic acid, copper, phenylalanine, sea cucumber, cartilage extracts, L-histidine, beta-carotene, ginger, burdock, horsetail, and Chinese herbal combinations.

Identifying and avoiding food allergens may be helpful in some cases.[27] Adopting a vegetarian diet sometimes brings about improvement in mild RA.[28,29]

ULCERS

Principal Natural Treatments
Deglycyrrhizinated licorice

Other Natural Treatments
Rhubarb, *Aloe vera,* bioflavonoids, vitamin A, zinc, omega-3 fatty acids, vitamin C, vitamin B_6, vitamin E, selenium, glutamine

The highly concentrated acid produced by the stomach is quite capable of burning a hole through the tissue of the stomach and duodenum (part of the small intestine). That it usually does not do so is a tribute to the effectiveness of the methods that the body uses to protect itself. However, sometimes these protective mechanisms fail, and the ever-present acid begins to produce an ulcer.

Ulcer pain is caused by stomach acid coming into contact with unprotected tissue. Eating generally decreases ulcer pain temporarily because food neutralizes the acid. As soon as the food begins to be digested, the pain returns.

Conventional medical treatment for ulcers has gone through a slow revolution. A few decades ago, the prescribed response to ulcers was a bland diet—one low in spices and high in dairy products, which were believed to coat the stomach. However, eventually it was discovered that spicy foods are innocent and that milk itself is somewhat ulcer forming! The only other option at that time was surgery.

Next came antacids containing magnesium and aluminum (such as Maalox). However, these were seldom strong enough to allow the ulcer to heal fully. Ulcer treatment took a big step forward with the development of Tagamet (cimetidine), followed by Zantac, Pepcid, and others. These drugs dramatically lower the stomach's production of acid. Later, a new class of even more potent acid suppressers appeared, led by Prilosec (omeperazole).

When stomach acid is suppressed, ulcer pain rapidly diminishes and the ulcer heals. For a time, these drugs were regarded as the definitive answer to ulcers. This early enthusiasm began to fade when it became clear that ulcers frequently returned after the drugs were stopped. In the late 1980s, a new explanation for this problem began to surface. First regarded as a wacky theory, it has now become the accepted explanation.

We now believe that ulcers are caused by the bacteria *Helicobacter pylori*. Apparently, this previously ignored organism has the capacity to infect the stomach and, by so doing, to weaken the stomach lining. Only when antibiotics to kill *Helicobacter pylori* are combined with stomach acid suppressants do ulcers go away and stay away.

Principal Natural Treatments for Ulcers

The most famous supplement used for ulcer disease is a special form of licorice known as deglycyrrhizinated licorice (DGL). This form of licorice eliminates the portion of the herb that can cause serious side effects.

Head-to-head comparison studies involving as many as 100 participants and lasting for up to 2 years suggest that DGL is more effective than the drug Tagamet (cimetidine) at healing ulcers and keeping them from recurring.[1,2,3]

DGL is believed to improve the health of the stomach lining and promote the production of substances that defend against acid. However, DGL has not been shown to kill *Helicobacter pylori*. It probably must be taken continuously to prevent ulcers.

Some natural medicine authorities suggest that DGL may help prevent ulcers caused by medications such as anti-inflammatory drugs and steroids.[4] However, there is no evidence as yet that this is true.

The proper dosage of DGL is 760 to 1,420 mg chewed 20 minutes before meals. For unknown reasons, studies suggest that chewing is essential to achieve full benefit.

DGL tastes bad but is believed to be very safe, although extensive safety studies have not been performed. Side effects are rare. Safety in young children, pregnant or nursing women, and those with severe liver or kidney disease has not been established.

Warning: Because ulcers can be dangerous, medical supervision of treatment is essential.

Other Natural Treatments for Ulcers

The following natural treatments are widely recommended, but they have not been scientifically proven effective at this time.

Rhubarb and *Aloe vera* have been suggested as treatments for bleeding ulcers.[5] However, this condition is sufficiently dangerous that conventional medical treatment is far more appropriate.

Highly preliminary studies suggest that various bioflavonoids can inhibit the growth of *Helicobacter pylori*.[6] All fruits and vegetables provide bioflavonoids, but these substances can also be taken as supplements. The dosage depends on the type of bioflavonoid used. A typical dosage for citrus bioflavonoids is 500 mg 3 times daily.

Vitamin A, zinc, omega-3 fatty acids, vitamin C, vitamin B_6, vitamin E, selenium, and glutamine have also been suggested as aids to ulcer healing, but there is little to no scientific evidence that they are effective.

VARICOSE VEINS

Principal Natural Treatments
Horse chestnut, grape seed PCOs, gotu kola, bilberry
Other Natural Treatments
Butcher's broom, aortic glycosaminoglycans, collinsonia, calendula

Walking upright has given our leg veins a difficult task. Although they lack the strong muscular lining of arteries, they must constantly return a large volume of blood to the heart. The movements of the legs act as a pump to push the blood upward while flimsy valves stop gravity from pulling it back down.

However, over time these valves often begin to fail. The blood then begins to pool, stretching the vein wall and injuring its lining. This situation is called *venous insufficiency*. Typically, the legs begin to feel heavy, achy, and tired. When enough injury has occurred, the veins visibly dilate and the cosmetically unpleasant torturous vessels known as varicose veins appear.

For unknown reasons, venous insufficiency affects women about three times as often as men. Occupations involving prolonged standing also increase the incidence of venous insufficiency. Pregnancy and obesity do so as well because of the increase of pressure in the abdomen that makes it more difficult for the blood to flow upward.

Conventional medical treatment of venous insufficiency consists mainly of reducing weight, elevating the legs, and wearing elastic support hose. Unsightly damaged veins can be destroyed by injection therapy or be surgically removed.

Principal Natural Treatments for Varicose Veins

Why are some illnesses luckier than others? Next to prostate enlargement, varicose veins have the most extensive repetoire of scientifically researched herbal treatments: four herbal treatments widely used in Europe for venous insufficiency.

These herbs have much in common. All of them appear to work by strengthening the walls of veins and other vessels. They primarily relieve symptoms of aching and swelling, rather than visible varicose veins. However, it is thought (but not proven) that the regular use of these treatments can prevent visible varicose veins from developing.

Warning: Symptoms similar to those caused by varicose veins can actually be due to more dangerous conditions, such as phlebitis. Medical evaluation is necessary prior to self-treating with the natural supplements described here.

Horse Chestnut: The Best-Documented
Treatment for Varicose Veins

The most popular German herbal treatment for venous insufficiency is horse chestnut. Closely related to the Ohio buckeye, its spiny fruits contain a few large seeds known as horse chestnuts. Medical use of this herb dates back to nineteenth-century France, where extracts were used to treat hemorrhoids (which are really a form of varicose veins).

German scientific research into horse chestnut began in the 1960s and ultimately led to Germany's Commission E approving the herb for vein diseases of the legs. In 1995, this herb was the third most common prescription herb in Germany, after ginkgo and St. John's wort.

What Is the Scientific Evidence for Horse Chestnut?

The clinical scientific evidence for horse chestnut as a treatment for venous insufficiency is moderately strong. A total of 558 participants have been involved in double-blind studies.[1] One of the largest followed 212 people over a period of 40 days using a crossover design.[2] Participants initially received either horse chestnut or placebo and then were crossed over to the other treatment (without their knowledge) after 20 days. Horse chestnut treatment significantly reduced leg edema, pain, and sensation of heaviness when compared to placebo.

Another study compared the effectiveness of horse chestnut and compression stockings in 240 people over a course of 12 weeks.[3] Compression stockings worked faster to lessen swelling, but by 12 weeks the results were equivalent between the two treatments.

Unlike many herbs, the active ingredients in horse chestnut have been identified to a reasonable degree of certainty. They appear to be a complex of related chemicals known collectively as aescin. Aescin reduces the rate of fluid leakage from stressed and irritated vessel walls. We don't really know how it does this, but the most prominent theory proposes that aescin plugs leaking capillaries and also prevents the release of enzymes that break down collagen and open holes in capillary walls.[4]

Dosage

The proper dosage of horse chestnut is 250 to 313 mg twice daily of an extract concentrated to contain 16 to 20% aescin, thus providing a total daily aescin dose of about 100 mg. After good results have been achieved, a maintenance dose 50% lower will often suffice to keep symptoms under control. Horse chestnut must be taken in a controlled-release enteric-coated form to minimize stomach discomfort.

Safety Issues

After decades of wide usage in Germany, no reports of harmful effects due to properly prepared horse chestnut have been noted, even when it has been taken in large overdose.[5] In animal studies, both horse chestnut and aescin have been found to be very safe. Dogs and rats have been treated for 34 weeks with this herb without harmful effects. However, doses 50 times higher than normal can cause death in animals, and in Japan, where injectable forms are used, occasional serious reactions have been noted.[6]

In clinical studies of horse chestnut, no significant side effects have been reported, other than the usual occasional mild allergic reactions or gastrointestinal distress. However, all these studies involved controlled-release enteric-coated forms of horse chestnut. This allowed it to pass through the stomach without dissolving. Taking horse chestnut in a standard capsule may cause severe stomach upset.

Based on relatively theoretical evidence, horse chestnut is not recommended for those with serious kidney or liver disease, and it should not be combined with blood thinners, such as Coumadin (warfarin), Trental (pentoxi-fylline), and aspirin. Its safety in pregnancy and nursing has not been established. However, no risks are known in pregnancy, and some studies have enrolled pregnant women.[7]

Grape Seed PCOs: Reasonably Good Evidence That Can They Help

Grape seed contains high levels of special bioflavonoids called PCOs (procyanidolic oligomers) or sometimes OPCs (oligomeric proanthocyanidin complexes). Similar substances are found in pine bark, cranberry, bilberry, blueberry, hawthorn and other plants.

PCOs are interesting antioxidant chemicals that appear to have the ability to improve collagen (a type of strength-ening tissue found in many parts of the body), reduce capillary leakage, and control inflammation.[8–11] In Europe, grape seed PCOs are widely used to treat venous insuffi-ciency, varicose veins, easy bruising, and hemorrhoids.

What Is the Scientific Evidence for Grape Seed PCOs?

Controlled studies involving a total of about 400 partici-pants have found that PCOs provide significant benefit for varicose veins.[12,13,14]

For example, a double-blind study comparing PCOs against placebo in 92 individuals showed improvement in 75% of the treated group as compared to 41% in the con-trol group.[15]

Dosage

PCOs are generally taken at a dosage of 150 to 300 mg daily when used for varicose veins. Lower doses are some-times recommended as a daily antioxidant supplement.

Safety Issues

Extensive studies have shown PCOs to be nontoxic.[16] Side effects are rare and are limited to mild gastrointestinal distress. However, safety in young children, pregnant or nursing women, and those with severe liver or kidney disease has not been established. PCOs may have some anticoagulant properties when taken in high doses, and should be used only under medical supervision by individuals on blood-thinner drugs such as Coumadin (warfarin), Trental (pentoxifylline), and heparin.

Gotu Kola: Also Effective

Another reasonably well documented treatment for venous insufficiency is the tropical creeper gotu kola, which should not be confused with the caffeine-containing kola nut (used in original recipes for Coca-Cola).

In India and Indonesia, gotu kola has a long history of use in promoting wound healing, treating skin diseases, and slowing the progress of leprosy. It was also reputed to prolong life, increase energy, and promote sexual potency.[17] In the 1970s, Italian and other European researchers discovered that gotu kola can significantly improve symptoms of venous insufficiency, and it subsequently became a popular European treatment for this condition.

In practice, 4 weeks of treatment with gotu kola frequently produces welcome benefits in the discomfort of chronic venous insufficiency. The active ingredients in gotu kola are believed to be asiaticoside, asiatic acid madecassic acid, and madecassoside.[18]

What Is the Scientific Evidence for Gotu Kola?

There is significant scientific evidence for the effectiveness of gotu kola in varicose veins/venous insufficiency.

A vacuum suction chamber has been used in some gotu kola studies to evaluate the rate of fluid leakage in venous insufficiency. It produces swelling when applied to the skin of the ankle. When leg veins are leaking a lot of fluid, this swelling takes longer to disappear.

In one study of people with venous insufficiency, 2 weeks of treatment with gotu kola extracts was shown to reduce the time necessary for the swelling to disappear.[19]

Another study of double-blind design followed 87 people with varicose veins and compared the benefits of gotu kola at 60 mg and 30 mg daily against placebo.[20] The results showed improvements in both treated groups but greater improvement at the higher dose. This kind of dose responsiveness is generally taken as good evidence that a treatment is actually effective.

A double-blind study of 94 individuals with venous insufficiency of the lower limb compared the benefits of gotu kola extract at 120 mg daily and 60 mg daily against a placebo.[21] The results also showed a significant dose-related improvement in the treated groups in symptoms such as subjective heaviness, discomfort, and edema.

A 1992 review of all the gotu kola studies available concluded that gotu kola extract provides a dose-related improvement in venous insufficiency symptoms, reducing foot swelling, ankle edema, and fluid leakage from the veins.[22]

Dosage

The usual dosage of gotu kola is 20 to 40 mg 3 times daily of an extract standardized to contain 40% asiaticoside, 29 to 30% asiatic acid, 29 to 30% madecassic acid, and 1 to 2% madecassoside.

Safety Issues

Studies suggest that oral asiaticoside at a dosage of 1 g per kilogram body weight is safe.[23] This leaves a wide margin of safety, since standard daily doses of gotu kola provide about 2,000 times less asiatocoside for an average adult. Studies have also found that doses of 16 g per kilogram body weight of fresh gotu kola leaves are nontoxic,[24] and recent studies suggest that gotu kola extracts are not harmful to fetal development.[25]

The only reported side effect with gotu kola is rare allergic skin rash. Safety in pregnancy has not been established. However, as with horse chestnut, one gotu kola study did enroll pregnant women.[26] Safety in young children, nursing mothers, and individuals with severe liver or kidney disease has not been established.

Bilberry: May Be Useful

Although much more famous as a treatment for eye problems (see the discussion of bilberry under Night Vision), there is some evidence that this relative of the American blueberry may be useful in varicose veins as well.

In a placebo-controlled study that followed 60 people with varicose veins for 30 days, bilberry extract significantly decreased pain and swelling.[27] Similar results were seen in another 30-day double-blind trial involving 47 participants.[28]

Bilberry contains substances known as anthocyanosides that are closely related to grape seed PCOs. Like PCOs, they appear to strengthen connective tissue, such as the walls of veins.[29,30,31] The standard dosage of bilberry is 120 to 240 mg twice daily of an extract standardized to contain 25% anthocyanosides.

Bilberry is a food and as such is believed to be quite safe. Enormous quantities have been administered to rats without toxic effects.[32] One study of 2,295 people given bilberry extract showed a 4% incidence of side effects, such as mild digestive distress, skin rashes, and drowsiness.[33] However, safety in young children, pregnant or nursing women, and those with severe liver or kidney disease has not been established. Bilberry may interfere with blood clotting when taken in high doses, and individuals on blood-thinning drugs, such as Coumadin (warfarin),

Trental (pentoxifylline), and heparin, should use bilberry only under medical supervision.

Other Natural Treatments for Varicose Veins

The following natural treatments are widely recommended for varicose veins, but they have not yet been scientifically proven effective.

Butcher's Broom

Butcher's broom is so named because its branches were a traditional source of broom straw used by butchers. This Mediterranean evergreen bush has a long history of traditional use in the treatment of urinary conditions. Recent European interest has focused on the possible value of butcher's broom in the treatment of hemorrhoids and varicose veins, although there is as yet no more than preliminary evidence that it is effective.

Butcher's broom is standardized to its ruscogenin content. A typical oral dose should supply 50 to 100 mg of ruscogenins daily.

Butcher's broom is believed to be safe when used as directed, although detailed studies have not been performed. Noticeable side effects are rare. However, safety in young children, pregnant or nursing women, and those with severe liver or kidney disease has not been established.

Aortic Glycosaminoglycans

A preparation made from the blood vessels of cows, known as aortic glycosaminoglycans, has been used in Italy as a remedy for varicose veins. Although it is said to be highly effective, the scientific evidence is not yet strong.[34,35,36]

The typical dosage is 100 mg daily. Aortic glycosaminoglycans are believed to be safe because they are widely found in foods. However, safety in young children, pregnant or nursing women, and those with severe liver or kidney disease has not been established.

Collinsonia

The herb collinsonia, or stone root, has a long traditional history of use as a treatment for varicose veins and hemorrhoids, but it has not been scientifically evaluated to any meaningful extent. The dosage varies with the preparation.

Calendula

A cream made from the herb calendula is said to be somewhat cosmetically helpful in varicose veins, although there is little evidence that this is true.

Notes

Acne
1. Pohit J, et al. Zinc status of acne vulgaris patients. *J Appl Nutr* 37(1): 18–25, 1985.
2. Amer M, et al. Serum zinc in acne vulgaris. *Int J Dermat* 21: 481, 1982.
3. Michaëlsson G, et al. Serum zinc and retinol-binding protein in acne. *Br J Dermatol* 96(3): 283–286, 1977.
4. Michaëlsson G and Ljunghall K. Patients with dermatitis herpetiformis, acne, psoriasis and Darier's disease have low epidermal zinc concentrations. *Acta Dermatovenereol (Stockh)* 70(4): 304–308, 1990.
5. Lidën S, et al. Clinical evaluation of acne. *Acta Dermatovenereol (Stockh)* 89(Suppl.): 49–52, 1980.
6. Dreno B, et al. Low doses of zinc gluconate for inflammatory acne. *Acta Dermatovenereol (Stockh)* 69(6): 541–543, 1989.
7. Verma KC, et al. Oral zinc sulfate therapy in acne vulgaris: a double-blind trial. *Acta Dermatovenereol (Stockh)* 60: 337, 1980.
8. Weimar VM, et al. Zinc sulfate in acne vulgaris. *Arch Dermatol* 114(12): 1776–1778, 1978.
9. Göransson K, et al. Oral zinc in acne vulgaris: a clinical and methodological study. *Acta Dermatovenereol (Stockh)* 58(5): 443–448, 1978.
10. Hillström L, Pettersson L, Hellbe L, et al. Comparison of oral treatment with zinc sulphate and placebo in acne vulgaris. *Br J Dermatol* 97(6): 679–684, 1977.
11. Michaëlsson G, Johlin L, and Ljunghall K. A double-blind study of the effect of zinc and oxytetracycline in acne vulgaris. *Br J Dermatol* 97(5): 561–566, 1977.
12. Cunliffe WJ, et al. A double-blind trial of a zinc sulphate/citrate complex and tetracycline in the treatment of acne vulgaris. *Br J Dermatol* 101(3): 321–325, 1979.

Allergies
1. Mittman P. Randomized, double-blind study of freeze-dried *Urtica dioica* in the treatment of allergic rhinitis. *Planta Medica* 56: 44–47, 1990.
2. Middleton E Jr, et al. The effects of citrus flavonoids on human basophil and neutrophil function. *Planta Medica* 53: 325–328, 1987.
3. Amellal M, Bronner C, Briancon F, et al. Inhibition of mast cell histamine release by flavonoids and bioflavonoids. *Planta Medica* 51: 16–20, 1985.
4. Gábor M. Anti-inflammatory and anti-allergic properties of flavonoids. *Prog Clin Biol Res* 213: 471–480, 1986.
5. Middleton E Jr. Effect of flavonoids on basophil histamine release and other secretory systems. *Prog Clin Biol Res* 213: 493–506, 1986.
6. Ogasawara H and Middleton E Jr. Effect of selected flavonoids on histamine release (HR) and hydrogen peroxide (H_2O_2) generation by human leukocytes. *J Allergy Clin Immunol* 75: 184, 1985.

7. Middleton E Jr and Drzewiecki G. Flavonoid inhibition of human basophil histamine release stimulated by various agents. *Biochem Pharmacol* 33(21): 3333, 1984.

8. Pearce FL, et al. Mucosal mast cells III. Effect of quercetin and other flavonoids on antigen-induced histamine secretion from rat intestinal mast cells. *J Allergy Clin Immunol* 73: 819–823, 1984.

9. Middleton E Jr, Drzewiecki G, and Krishnarao D. Quercetin: an inhibitor of antigen-induced human basophil histamine release. *J Immunol* 127(2): 546–550, 1981.

10. Yoshimoto T, et al. Flavonoids: potent inhibitors of arachidonate 5-lipoxygenase. *Biochem Biophys Res Commun* 116: 612–618, 1983.

11. Bucca C, et al. Effect of vitamin C on histamine bronchial responsiveness of patients with allergic rhinitis. *Ann Allergy* 65: 311–314, 1990.

12. Bellioni P, et al. La provocazione istaminica in soggetti allergici. Il ruolo dell'acido ascorbico. *Eur Rev Med Pharmacol Sci* 9: 419–422, 1987.

13. Fortner BR Jr, et al. The effect of ascorbic acid on cutaneous and nasal response to histamine and allergen. *J Allergy Clin Immunol* 69(6): 484–488, 1982.

Alzheimer's Disease

1. Stoppe G, et al. Prescribing practice with cognition enhancers in outpatient care: are there differences regarding type of dementia? Results of a representative survey in lower Saxony, Germany. *Pharmacopsychiatry* 29(4): 150–155, 1996.

2. Kleijnen J and Knipschild P. Ginkgo biloba. *Lancet* 340: 1136–1139, 1992.

3. Hofferberth B. The efficacy of EGb 761 in patients with senile dementia of the Alzheimer type, a double-blind, placebo-controlled study on different levels of investigation. *Hum Psychopharmacol* 9: 215–222, 1994.

4. Kanowski S, et al. Proof of efficacy of the *Ginkgo biloba* special extract EGb 761 in outpatients suffering from mild to moderate primary degenerative dementia of the Alzheimer type or multi-infarct dementia. *Pharmacopsychiatry* 29: 47–56, 1996.

5. Schulz V, et al. Rational phytotherapy. New York: Springer-Verlag, 1998: 46–47.

6. LeBars PL, et al. A placebo-controlled, double-blind, randomized trial of an extract of *Ginkgo biloba* for dementia. *JAMA* 278: 1327–1332, 1997.

7. Schulz V, et al., 1998: 43.

8. Schulz V, et al., 1998: 41.

9. De Feudis FV. *Ginkgo biloba* extract (EGb 761): Pharmacological activity and clinical applications. Paris: Elsevier, 1991: 143–146.

10. Rosenblatt M and Mindel J. Spontaneous hyphema associated with ingestion of *Ginkgo biloba* extract. *N Engl J Med* 336(15): 1108, 1997.

11. Rowin J and Lewis SL. Spontaneous bilateral subdural hematomas associated with chronic *Ginkgo biloba* ingestion. *Neurology* 46: 1775–1776, 1996.

12. Cenacchi T, et al. Cognitive decline in the elderly: a double-blind, placebo-controlled multicenter study on efficacy of phosphatidylserine administration. *Aging* 5: 123–133, 1993.

13. Crook T, et al. Effects of phosphatidylserine in age-associated memory impairment. *Neurology* 41(5): 644–649, 1991.

14. Delwaide PJ, et al. Double-blind randomized controlled study of phosphatidylserine in senile demented patients. *Acta Neurol Scand* 73(2): 136–140, 1986.

15. Engel RR, et al. Double-blind cross-over study of phosphatidylserine vs. placebo in subjects with early cognitive deterioration of the Alzheimer type. *Eur Neuropsychopharmacol* 2: 149–155, 1992.

16. Fagioli S, et al. Phosphatidylserine administration during postnatal development improves memory in adult mice. *Neurosci Lett* 101(2): 229–233, 1989.

17. Funfgeld E, et al. Double-blind study with phosphatidylserine (PS) in Parkinsonian patients with senile dementia of Alzheimer's type (SDAT). *Prog Clin Biol Res* 317: 1235–1246, 1989.

18. Crook T, et al. Effects of phosphatidylserine in Alzheimer's disease. *Psychopharmacol Bull* 28: 161–166, 1992.

19. Amaducci L, et al. Phosphatidylserine in the treatment of Alzheimer's disease: results of a multicenter study. *Psychopharmacol Bull* 24(1): 130–134, 1988.

20. Villardita C, et al. Multicenter clinical trial of brain phosphatidylserine in elderly patients with intellectual deterioration. *Clin Trials J* 24(1): 84–89, 1987.

21. Palmieri G, et al. Double-blind controlled trial of phosphatidylserine in patients with senile mental deterioration. *Clin Trials J* 24(1): 73–83, 1987.

22. Van den Besselaar AM. Phosphatidylethanolamine and phosphatidylserine synergistically promote heparin's anticoagulant effect. *Blood Coagul Fibrinolysis* 6: 239–244, 1995.

23. Salvioli G and Neri M. L-acetylcarnitine treatment of mental decline in the elderly. *Drugs Exp Clin Res* 20(4): 169–176, 1994.

24. Calvani M, Carta A, Caruso G, et al. Action of acetyl-L-carnitine in neurodegeneration and Alzheimer's disease. *Ann NY Acad Sci* 663: 483–486, 1992.

25. Spagnoli A, Lucca U, Menasce G, et al. Long-term acetyl-L-carnitine treatment in Alzheimer's disease. *Neurology* 41(11): 1726–1732, 1991.

26. Passeri et al. Acetyl-L-carnitine in the treatment of mildly demeneted elderly patients. *Int J Clin Pharmacol Res* 10: 75–79, 1990.

27. Sano et al. Double-blind parallel design pilot study of acetyl levocarnitine in patients with Alzheimer's disease. *Arch Neurol* 49: 1137–1141, 1992.

28. Campi et al. Selegiline versus L-acetylcarnitine in the treatment of Alzheimer-type dementia. *Clin Ther* 12: 306–314, 1990.

29. Garzya et al. Evaluation of the effects of L-acetylcarnitine on senile patients suffering from depression. *Drugs Exp Clin Res* 16: 101–106, 1990.

30. Vecchi et al. Methodology of a controlled clinical study for cerebral aging evaluation. *Int J Clin Pharamcol Res* 10: 145–152, 1990.

31. Rai et al. Double-blind placebo-controlled study of acetyl-L-carnitine in patients with Alzheimer's dementia. *Curr Med Res Opin* 11: 638–647, 1990.

32. Bonavita E. Study of the efficacy and tolerability of L-acetylcarnitine therapy in the senile brain. *Int J Clin Pharmacol Ther Toxicol* 24: 511–516, 1986.

33. Bella R, Biondi R, Raffaele R, et al. Effect of acetyl-L-carnitine on geriatric patients suffering from dysthymic disorders. *Int J Clin Pharmacol Res* 10: 355–360, 1990.

34. Spagnoli A, Lucca U, Menasce G, et al., 1991.

35. Thal LJ, Carta A, Clarke WR, et al. A 1-year multicenter placebo-controlled study of acetyl-L-carnitine in patients with Alzheimer's disease. *Neurology* 47: 705–711, 1996.

36. Goa KL, et al. L-carnitine—A preliminary review of its pharmacokinetics and its therapeutic use in ischemic cardiac disease and primary and secondary carnitine deficiencies in relationship to its role in fatty acid metabolism. *Drugs* 34: 1–24, 1987.

37. Sano M, Ernesto C, Thomas RG, et al. A controlled trial of selegiline, alpha-tocopherol, or both as treatment for Alzheimer's disease. *N Engl J Med* 336: 1216–1222, 1997.

Angina

1. Cacciatore L, et al. The therapeutic effect of L-carnitine in patients with exercise-induced stable angina: a controlled study. *Drugs Exp Clin Res* 17: 225–335, 1991.

2. Bartels GL, et al. Anti-ischaemic efficacy of L-propionylcarnitine—A promising novel metabolic approach to ischaemia? *Eur Heart J* 17(3): 414–420, 1996.

3. Kamikawa T, et al. Effects of coenzyme Q_{10} on exercise tolerance in chronic stable angina pectoris. *Am J Cardiol* 56: 247, 1985.

4. McLean RM. Magnesium and its therapeutic uses: a review. *Am J Med* 96: 63–76, 1994.

5. Ornish D, et al. Can lifestyle changes reverse coronary heart disease? *Lancet* 336: 129–133, 1990.

Anxiety

1. Meyer HJ, et al. Kawa-Pyrone-eine neuartige Substanzgruppe zentraler Muskel-relaxantien vom Typ des Mephenesins. *Klin Wochenschr* 44: 902–903, 1966.

2. Klohs MW, et al. A chemical and pharmacological investigation of *Piper methysticum forst. J Med Pharmacol Chem* 1: 95–103, 1959.

3. Bruggenmann F, et al. Die analgetische Wirkung der Kawa-Inhaltsstoffe Dihydrokawain und Dihydromethysticin. *Arzneimittelforschung* 13: 407–409, 1963.

4. Meyer HJ. Pharmakologie der Wirksamen Prinzipien des Kawa-Rhizoms (*Piper methysticum Forst*). *Arch Int Pharmacodyn Therapie* 138: 505–535, 1982.

5. Meyer HJ. Lokalanaesthetische Eigenschaften naturlicher Kawa-Pyrone. *Arzneimittelforschung* 42: 407, 1964.

6. Meyer HJ, et al., 1966.

7. Singh YN. Effects of kava on neuromuscular transmission and muscle contractility. *Ethnopharmacology* 7: 267–276, 1983.

8. Volz HP, et al. Kava-kava extract WS 1490 versus placebo in anxiety disorders—A randomized placebo-controlled 25 week outpatient trial. *Pharmacopsychiatry* 30(1): 1–5, 1997.

9. Kinzler E, et al. Effect of a special kava extract in patients with anxiety-, tension-, and excitation states of nonpsychotic genesis. Double-blind study with placebos over 4 weeks. *Arzneimittelforschung* 41(6): 584–588, 1991.

10. Warnecke G, et al. Wirksamkeit von Kawa-Kawa-Extract beim klimakterischen Syndrom. *Z Phytother* 11: 81–86, 1990.

11. Warnecke G. Psychosomatic dysfunctions in the female climacteric. Clinical effectiveness and tolerance of kava extract WS 1490 *Fortschr Med* 109(4): 119–122, 1991.

12. Woelk H, et al. Behandlung von Angst-Patienten. *Z Allg* 69: 271–277, 1993.

13. Jussofie A, Schmiz A, and Hiemke C. Kavapyrone enriched extract from *Piper methysticum* as modulator of the GABA binding site in different regions of rat brain. *Psychopharmacology* 116: 469–474, 1994.

14. Schulz V, et al. Rational phytotherapy. New York: Springer-Verlag, 1998.

15. Schulz V, et al., 1998.

16. Schulz V, et al., 1998.

17. Norton SA, et al. Kava dermopathy. *Am Acad Dermatol* 31(1): 89–97, 1994.

18. Munte TF, et al. Effects of oxazepam and an extract of kava roots (*Piper methysticum*) on event-related potentials in a word recognition task. *Neuropsychobiology* 27(1): 46–53, 1993.

19. Heinze HJ, et al. Pharmacopsychological effects of oxazepam and kava extract in a visual search paradigm assessed with event-related potentials. *Pharmacopsychiatry* 27(6): 224–230, 1994.

20. Herberg KW. Effect of Kava-Special Extract WS 1490 combined with ethyl alcohol on safety-relevant performance parameters. *Blutalkohol* 30(2): 96–105, 1993.

21. Cawte J. Parameters of kava used as a challenge to alcohol. *Aust N Z J Psychiatry* 20(1): 70–76, 1986.

22. Schulz V, et al. 1998: 72.

23. Duffield PH and Jamieson D. Development of tolerance to kava in mice. *Clin Exp Pharmacol Physiol* 18: 571–578, 1991.

24. Almeida JC and Grimsley EW. Coma from the health-food store: interaction between kava and alprazolam. *Ann Intern Med:* 1996.

25. Kohnen R, et al. The effects of valerian, propranolol, and their combination on activation, performance and mood of healthy volunteers under social stress conditions. *Pharmacopsychiatry* 21: 447–448, 1988.

Asthma

1. Shivpuri DN, et al. Treatment of asthma with an alcoholic extract of *Tylphora indica:* a crossover, double-blind study. *Ann Allergy* 30: 407–412, 1972.

2. Shivpuri DN, et al. A crossover double-blind study on *Tylophora indica* in the treatment of asthma and allergic rhinitis. *J Allergy* 43: 145–150, 1969.

3. Gupta S, et al. *Tylphora indica* in bronchial asthma—A double-blind study. *Ind J Med Res* 69: 981–989, 1979.

4. Hatch GE. Asthma, inhaled oxidants, and dietary antioxidants. *Am J Clin Nutr* 61(Suppl. 3): 625S–630S, 1995.

5. Bielory L and Gandhi R. Asthma and vitamin C. *Ann Allergy* 73(2): 89–96, 1994.

6. Wright J. Vitamin B$_{12}$: Powerful protection against asthma. *Int Clin Nutr Rev* 9(4): 185–188, 1989.

7. Collipp PJ. Pyridoxine treatment of childhood bronchial asthma. *Ann Allergy* 35: 93–97, 1975.

8. Sur S, Camara M, Buchmeier A, et al. Double-blind trial of pyridoxine (vitamin B$_6$) in the treatment of steroid-dependent asthma. *Ann Allergy* 70: 147–152, 1993.

9. Dry J and Vincent D. Effects of a fish oil diet on asthma: results of a one-year double-blind study. *Int Arch Allergy Immunol* 95: 156–157, 1991.

10. Stenius-Aarniala B, Aro A, Hakaulinen A, et al. Evening primrose oil and fish oil are ineffective as supplementary treatment of bronchial asthma. *Ann Allergy* 62(6): 534–547, 1989.

11. Picado C, et al. Effects of a fish oil enriched diet on aspirin intolerant asthmatic patients: a pilot study. *Thorax* 43(2): 93–97, 1988.

12. Arm J, et al. The effects of dietary supplementation with fish oil on asthmatic responses to antigen. *J Clin Allergy* 81: 183, 1988.

13. Stenius-Aarniala B, et al. Symptomatic effects of evening primrose oil, fish oil, and olive oil in patients with bronchial asthma (Abstract). *Ann Allergy* 55: 330, 1985.

14. Thien FC, et al. Fish oils and asthma—A fishy story? *Med J Aust* 164: 135–136, 1996.

15. Arm JP, Thien FC, and Lee TH. Leukotrienes, fish oil, and asthma. *Allergy Proc* 15: 129–134, 1994.

16. Lee TH and Arm JP. Prospects for modifying the allergic response by fish oil diets. *Clin Allergy* 16(2): 89–100, 1986.

17. Monteleone CA and Sherman AR. Nutrition and asthma. *Arch Intern Med* 157: 23–24, 1997.

18. Rolla G, et al. Magnesium attenuates methacholine-induced bronchoconstriction in asthmatics. *Magnesium* 6(4): 201–204, 1987.

Atherosclerosis

1. Stephens NG, Parsons A, Schofield PM, et al. Randomized controlled trial of vitamin E in patients with coronary disease: Cambridge Heart Antioxidant Study (CHAOS). *Lancet* 347: 781–786, 1996.

2. Rapola JM, Virtamo J, Ripatti S, et al. Randomized trial of alpha-tocopherol and beta-carotene supplements on incidence of major coronary events in men with previous myocardial infarction. *Lancet* 349: 1715–1720, 1997.

3. Albanes D, Heinonen OP, Huttunen JK, et al. Effects of alpha-tocopherol and beta-carotene supplements on cancer incidence in the Alpha-Tocopherol Beta-Carotene Cancer Prevention Study. *Am J Clin Nutr* 62(Suppl.): 1427S–1430S, 1995.

4. Losonczy KG, Harris TB, and Havlik RJ. Vitamin E and vitamin C supplement use and risk of all-cause and coronary heart disease mortality in older persons: the established populations for epidemiologic studies of the elderly. *Am J Clin Nutr* 64: 190–196, 1996.

5. Rimm EB, Stampfer MJ, Ascherio A, et al. Vitamin E consumption and the risk of coronary heart disease in men. *N Engl J Med* 328(20): 1450–1456, 1993.

6. Stampfer M, Hennekens C, Manson J, et al. Vitamin E consumption and the risk of coronary heart disease in women. *N Engl J Med* 328: 1444–1449, 1993.

7. Jialal I and Fuller CJ. Effect of vitamin E, vitamin C, and beta-carotene on LDL oxidation and atherosclerosis. *Can J Cardiol* 1(Suppl. G): 97G–103G, 1995.

8. Morel DW, de la Llera-Moya M, and Friday KE. Treatment of cholesterol-fed rabbits with dietary vitamins E and C inhibits lipoprotein oxidation but not development of atherosclerosis. *J Nutr* 124: 2123–2130, 1994.

9. Calzada C, Bruckdorfer K, and Rice-Evans C. The influence of antioxidant nutrients on platelet function in healthy volunteers. *Atherosclerosis* 128(1): 97–105, 1997.

10. Albanes D, Heinonen OP, Huttunen JK, et al. 1995.

11. Bellizzi MC, Franklin MF, Duthie GG, et al. Vitamin E and coronary heart disease: the European paradox. *Eur J Clin Nutr* 48: 822–831, 1994.

12. Steiner M, Glantz M, and Lekos A. Vitamin E plus aspirin compared with aspirin alone in patients with transient ischemic attacks. *Am J Clin Nutr* 62(Suppl.): 1381S–1384S, 1995.

13. Ness AR. Vitamin C and cardiovascular disease. *Nutr Rep* 15(3): 1997.

14. Simon JA. Vitamin C and cardiovascular disease: a review. *J Am Coll Nutr* 11(2): 107–125, 1992.

15. Trout DL. Vitamin C and cardiovascular risk factors. *Am J Clin Nutr* 53: 322S–325S, 1991.

16. Kohlmeier L and Hastings SB. Epidemiologic evidence of a role of carotenoids in cardiovascular disease prevention. *Am J Clin Nutr* 62(Suppl.): 1370S–1376S, 1995.

17. Albanes D, et al. Alpha-Tocopherol, Beta-Carotene Cancer Prevention Study Group. The effect of vitamin E and beta-carotene on the incidence of lung cancer and other cancers in male smokers. *N Engl J Med* 330: 1029–1035, 1994.

18. Rapola JM, Virtamo J, Ripatti S, et al., 1997.

19. Rapola JM, Virtamo J, Haukka JK, et al. Effect of vitamin E and beta-carotene on the incidence of angina pectoris. *JAMA* 275(9): 693–698, 1996.

20. Kohlmeier L and Hastings SB., 1995.

21. White WS, et al. Pharmacokinetics of beta-carotene and canthaxanthin after individual and combined doses by human subjects. *J Am Coll Nutr* 13: 665–671, 1994.

22. Efendi JL, et al. The effect of the aged garlic extract, "Kyolic," on the development of experimental atherosclerosis. *Atherosclerosis* 132(1): 37–42, 1997.

23. Schulz V, et al. Rational phytotherapy. New York: Springer-Verlag, 1998: 112.

24. Breithaupt-Grogler K, et al. Protective effect of chronic garlic intake on the elastic properties of the aorta in the elderly. *Circulation* 96(7): 2649–2655, 1997.

25. Dyerberg J. N-3 fatty acids and coronary artery disease: potentials and problems. *Omega-3, Lipoproteins Atherosclerosis* 27: 251–258, 1996.

26. Harris WS. N-3 fatty acids and serum lipoproteins: human studies. *Am J Clin Nutr* 65(Suppl): 1645S–1654S, 1997.

27. Dyerberg J., 1996.

28. Prichard BN, et al. Fish oils and cardiovascular disease. *BMJ* 310: 819–820, 1995.

29. Stone NJ. From the Nutrition Committee of the American Heart Association. Fish consumption, fish oil, lipids, and coronary heart disease. *Am J Clin Nutr* 65: 1083–1086, 1997.

30. Harris WS. Dietary fish oil and blood lipids. *Curr Opin Lipidol* 7: 3–7, 1996.

31. Harris WS., 1997.

32. Laurora G, et al. Control of the progress of arteriosclerosis in high risk subjects treated with mesoglycan: measuring the intima media. *Minerva Cardioangiol* 46(3): 41–47, 1998.

33. Laurora G, Cesarone MR, De Sanctis MT, et al. Delayed arteriosclerosis progression in high-risk subjects treated with mesoglycan. Evaluation of intima-media thickness. *J Cardiovasc Surg (Torino)* 34(4): 313–318, 1993.

34. Tanganelli P, Bianciardi G, Carducci A, et al. Updating on in-vivo and in-vitro effects of heparin and other glycosaminoglycans (mesoglycan) on arterial endothelium: a morphometrical study. *Int J Tissue React* 14(3): 149–153, 1992.

35. Kubow S. Lipid oxidation products in food and atherogenesis. *Nutr Rev* 51(2): 33–39, 1993.

36. Kromhout D, et al. Alcohol, fish, fibre and antioxidant vitamins intake do not explain population differences in coronary heart disease mortality. *Int J Epidemiol* 25: 753–759, 1996.

37. Pietinen P, et al. Intake of fatty acids and risk of coronary heart disease in a cohort of Finnish men: the Alpha-Tocopherol, Beta-Carotene Cancer Prevention Study. *Am J Epidemiol* 145(10): 876–887, 1997.

38. Pearson TA. Alcohol and heart disease. *Circulation* 94(11): 3023–3025, 1996.

39. Rimm EB and Ellison RC. Alcohol in the Mediterranean diet. *Am J Clin Nutr* 61(Suppl.): 1378S–1382S, 1995.

40. Hammar N, Romelsjo A, and Alfredsson L. Alcohol consumption, drinking pattern and acute myocardial infarction: a case reference study based on the Swedish twin register. *J Intern Med* 241(2): 125–131, 1997.

41. Camargo CA Jr, et al. Moderate alcohol consumption and risk for angina pectoris or myocardial infarction in U.S. male physicians. *Ann Intern Med* 126(5): 372–375, 1997.

42. Kawachi K, Colditz GA, and Stone CB. Does coffee drinking increase the risk of coronary heart disease? Results from a meta-analysis. *Br Heart J* 72: 269–275, 1994.

43. Willett WC, Stampfer MJ, Manson JA, et al. Coffee consumption and coronary heart disease in women: a ten-year follow-up. *JAMA* 275(6): 458–462, 1996.

44. Nyg RD, et al. Coffee consumption and plasma total homocysteine: the Hordaland Homocysteine Study. *Am J Clin Nutr* 65: 136–143, 1997.

Attention Deficit Disorder

1. Kleijnen J and Knipschild P. Niacin and vitamin B_6 in mental functioning: a review of controlled trials in humans. *Biol Psychiatry* 29(9): 931–941, 1991.

Benign Prostatic Hyperplasia

1. Emili E, et al. Clinical trial of a new drug for treating hypertrophy of the prostate (Permixon). Urologia 50: 1042–1048, 1983.

2. Champault G, et al. A double-blind trial of an extract of the plant *Serenoa repens* in benign prostatic hyperplasia. *Br J Clin Pharmacol* 18(3): 461–462, 1984.

3. Tasca A, et al. Treatment of obstructive symptomatology caused by prostatic adenoma with an extract of *Serenoa repens.* Double-blind clinical study vs. placebo. *Minerva Urol Nefrol* 37(1): 87–91, 1985.

4. Boccafoschi S et al. Comparison of *Serenoa repens* extract with placebo by controlled clinical trial in patients with prostatic adenomatosis. *Urologia* 50: 1257–1268, 1983.

5. Smith RH, et al. The value of Permixon in benign prostatic hypertrophy *Br J Urol* 58:36–40, 1986.

6. Descotes JL, et al. Placebo-controlled evaluation of the efficacy and tolerability of Permixon in benign prostatic hyperplasia after exclusion of placebo responders. *Clin Drug Invest* 9: 291–297, 1995.

7. Mattei FM, et al. *Serenoa repens* extract in the medical treatment of benign prostatic hypertrophy. Urologia 55: 547–552, 1988.

8. Carraro J, et al. Comparison of phytotherapy (Permixon) with finasteride in the treatment of benign prostate hyperplasia: a randomized international study of 1,098 patients. *Prostate* 29(4): 231–240, 1996.

9. Plosker GL, et al., *Serenoa repens* (Permixon). A review of its pharmacology and therapeutic efficacy in benign prostatic hyperplasia. *Drugs Aging* 9(5): 379–395, 1996.

10. Plosker GL, et al., 1996.

11. Bach D, et al. Phytopharmaceutical and synthetic agents in the treatment of benign prostatic hyperplasia (BPH). *Phytomedicine* 3(4): 309–313, 1997.

12. Duvia R, et al. Advances in the phytotherapy of prostatic hypertrophy. *Med Praxis* 4: 143–148, 1983.

13. Schulz V, et al. Rational phytotherapy. New York: Springer-Verlag, 1998: 233.

14. Schulz V, et al., 1998.

15. Dathe G and Schmid H. Phytotherapy of benign prostate hyperplasia with *Serenoa repens* extract (Permixon(R)). *Urologe Ausg B* 31(5): 220–223, 1991.

16. ESCOP monographs. Fascicule 2: *Urticae radix.* Exeter, UK: European Scientific Cooperative on Phytotherapy, 1997: 4.

17. ESCOP monographs, 1997.

18. Schulz V, et al., 1998: 229.

19. Berges RR, et al., Randomised, placebo-controlled, double-blind clinical trial of beta-sitosterol in patients with benign prostatic hyperplasia. *Lancet* 345: 1529–1532, 1995.

20. Schulz V, et al., 1998: 231.

21. Berges RR, et al., 1995.

22. Buck AC, et al. Treatment of outflow tract obstruction due to benign prostatic hyperplasia with the pollen extract, Cernilton: a double-blind placebo-controlled study. *Br J Urol* 66(4): 398–404, 1990.

23. Schultz V., et al., 1998: 229–230.

Bladder Infection

1. Sobota AE. Inhibition of bacterial adherence by cranberry juice: potential use for the treatment of urinary tract infections. *J Urol* 131(5): 1013–1016, 1984.

2. Schmidt DR, et al. An examination of the anti-adherence activity of cranberry juice on urinary and nonurinary bacterial isolates. *Microbios* 55: 173–181, 224–225, 1998.

3. Zafriri D, et al. Inhibitory activity of cranberry juice on adherence of type 1 and type P fimbriated *Escherichia coli* to eucaryotic cells. *Antimicrob Agents Chemother* 33(1): 92–98, 1989.

4. Howell A, et al. Letter. *N Engl J Med* 339: 1085, 1998.

5. Schaefer AJ. Recurrent urinary tract infections in the female patient. *Urology* 32 (Suppl.): 12–15, 1988.

6. Avorn J, et al. Reduction of bacteriuria and pyuria after ingestion of cranberry juice. *JAMA* 271(10): 751–754, 1994.

7. Frohne V, et al. Untersuchungen zur Frage der harndesifizierenden Wirkungen von Barentraubenblatt-extracten. *Planta Med* 18: 1–25, 1970. As cited in ESCOP, Fascicule 5: *Uvae Ursi Folium* (bearberry leaf). Exeter, UK: European Scientific Cooperative on Phytotherapy, 1997: 2.

8. ESCOP monographs, 1997.

9. Schulz V, et al. Rational phytotherapy. New York: Springer-Verlag, 1998: 223.

10. ESCOP monographs, 1997.

11. Kedzia B, et al. Antibacterial action of urine containing arbutin metabolic products. *Med Dosw Mikrobiol* 27: 305–314, 1975.

12. Larsson B, et al. Prophylactic effect of UVA-E in women with recurrent cystitis: a preliminary report. *Curr Ther Res* 53: 441–443, 1993.

13. ESCOP monographs, 1997.

14. Tyler V. Herbs of choice. New York: Pharmaceutical Production Press, 1994: 79.

15. Schulz V, et al., 1998: 224.

16. Nowak AK, et al., Darkroom hepatitis after exposure to hydroquinone. *Lancet* 345: 1187, 1995.

17. U.S. Environmental Protection Agency. Extremely hazardous substances: Superfund chemical profiles. Park Ridge NJ: Noyes Data Corporation, 1988: 1906–1907.

18. Lewis RJ. Sax's dangerous properties of industrial materials, 8th ed. New York: Van Nostrand Reinhold, 1989: 1906–1907.

19. Schulz V, et al. 1998: 223.

20. ESCOP monographs, 1997.

Cancer Prevention: Reducing the Risk

1. Longo D. Approach to the patient with cancer (ch. 81) in Harrison's principles of internal medicine, 14th ed. New York: McGraw-Hill, 1998.

2. Welland D. 15 cancer-preventing strategies that stack the odds in your favor. *Environ Nutr* 21(3): 1, 1998.

3. Osborne M, et al. Cancer prevention. *Lancet* 349(Suppl. 2): SII27–SII30, 1997.

4. Heinonen OP, et al. Prostate cancer and supplementation with alpha-tocopherol and beta-carotene: incidence and mortality in a controlled trial. *J Natl Cancer Inst* 90(6): 440–446, 1998.

5. White E, et al. Relationship between vitamin and calcium supplement use and colon cancer. *Cancer Epidemiol Biomarkers Prev* 6(10): 769–774, 1997.

6. Macready N. Vitamins associated with lower colon-cancer risk. *Lancet* 350: 9089, 1997.

7. Losonczy KG, Harris TB, and Havlik RJ. Vitamin E and vitamin C supplement use and risk of all-cause and coronary heart disease mortality in older persons: the established populations for epidemiologic studies of the elderly. *Am J Clin Nutr* 64: 190–196, 1996.

8. Bostick RM, Potter JD, McKenzie DR, et al. Reduced risk of colon cancer with high intake of vitamin E: the Iowa Women's Health Study. *Cancer Res* 53: 4230–4237, 1993.

9. Zheng W, Sellers TA, Doyle TJ, et al. Retinol, antioxidant vitamins, and cancer of the upper digestive tract in a prospective cohort study of postmenopausal women. *Am J Epidemiol* 142: 955–960, 1995.

10. Esteve J, et al. Diet and cancers of the larynx and hypopharynx: the IARC multicenter study in southwestern Europe. *Cancer Causes Control* 7: 240–252, 1996.

11. Albanes D, Heinonen OP, Huttunen JK, et al. Effects of alpha-tocopherol and beta-carotene supplements on cancer incidence in the Alpha-Tocopherol Beta-Carotene Cancer Prevention Study. *Am J Clin Nutr* 62(Suppl.): 1427S–1430S, 1995.

12. Chen J, Geissler C, Parpia B, et al. Antioxidant status and cancer mortality in China. *Int J Epidemiol* 21: 625–635, 1992.

13. Ocke M, Bueno-deo-Mesquita H, Feskens E, et al. Repeated measurements of vegetables, fruits, beta-carotene, and vitamins C and E in relation to lung cancer. *Am J Epidemiol* 145(4): 358–365, 1997.

14. Bellizzi MC, Franklin MF, Duthie GG, et al. Vitamin E and coronary heart disease: the European paradox. *Eur J Clin Nutr* 48: 822–831, 1994.

15. Albanes D, Heinonen OP, Huttunen JK, et al., 1995.

16. National Research Council. Diet and health: implications for reducing chronic risk. Washington DC: National Academy Press, 1989: 376–379.

17. Clark LC, Combs GF Jr, Turnbull BW, et al. Effects of selenium supplementation for cancer prevention in patients with carcinoma of the skin. *JAMA* 276(24): 1957–1963, 1996.

18. Fan AM, et al. Selenium: nutritional, toxicological and clinical aspects. *West J Med* 153: 160–167, 1990.

19. Steinmetz KA, et al. Vegetables, fruit and colon cancer in the Iowa Women's Health Study. *Am J Epidemiol* 139(1): 1–13, 1994.

20. Sumiyoshi H. New pharmacological activities of garlic and its constituents. *Nippon Yakurigaku Zasshi* 110(Suppl. 1): 93P–97P, 1997.

21. Agarwal KC. Therapeutic actions of garlic constituents. *Med Res Rev* 16(1): 111–124, 1996.

22. Popov I, et al. Antioxidant effects of aqueous garlic extract, 1st communication: direct detection using photochemoluminescence. *Arzneimittelforschung Drug Res* 44(1): 602–604, 1994.

23. Torok B, et al. Effectiveness of garlic on radical activity in radical generating systems. *Arzneimittelforschung Drug Res* 44(1): 608–611, 1994.

24. Das T, et al. Modification of clastogenicity of three known clastogens by garlic extract in mice in vivo. *Environ Mol Mutagen* 21(4): 383–388, 1993.

25. Ip C, et al. Efficacy of cancer prevention by high-selenium garlic is primarily dependent on the action of selenium. *Carcinogenesis* 16(11): 2649–2652, 1995.

26. Steinmetz KA and Potter JD. Vegetables, fruit, and cancer prevention: a review. *J Am Diet Assoc* 96(10): 1027–1039, 1996.

27. Ziegler RG. A review of epidemiologic evidence that carotenoids reduce the risk of cancer. *J Nutr* 119: 116–122, 1989.

28. Flagg EW, Coates RJ, and Greenberg RS. Epidemiologic studies of antioxidants and cancer. *J Am Coll Nutr* 14(5): 419–427, 1995.

29. Vena JE, Graham S, Freudenheim J, et al. Diet in the epidemiology of bladder cancer in western New York. *Nutr Cancer* 18(3): 255–264, 1992.

30. Rock CL, Saxe GA, Ruffin MT IV, et al. Carotenoids, vitamin A, and estrogen receptor status in breast cancer. *Nutr Cancer* 25(3): 281–296, 1996.

31. Zheng W, Sellers TA, Doyle TJ, et al., 1995.

32. Zheng W, Sellers TA, Doyle TJ, et al., 1995.

33. Santamaria L and Bianchi-Santamaria A. Carotenoids in cancer chemoprevention and therapeutic interventions. *J Nutr Sci Vitaminol (Tokyo) Spec* 321: 6, 1992.

34. Albanes D, Heinonen OP, Huttunen JK, et al., 1995.

35. Omenn GS, Goodman GE, Thornquist MD, et al. Effects of a combination of beta-carotene and vitamin A on lung cancer and cardiovascular disease. *N Engl J Med* 334: 1150–1155, 1996.

36. Hennekens CH, Buring JE, Manson JAE, et al. Lack of effect of long-term supplementation with beta-carotene on the incidence of malignant neoplasms and cardiovascular disease. *N Engl J Med* 334(18): 1145–1149, 1996.

37. White WS, et al. Pharmacokinetics of beta-carotene and canthaxanthin after individual and combined doses by human subjects. *J Am Coll Nutr* 13: 665–671, 1994.

38. Franceschi S, et al. Tomatoes and risk of digestive-tract cancers. *Int J Cancer* 59: 181–184, 1994.

39. Giovannucci E, Ascherio A, Rimm EB, et al. Intake of carotenoids and retinol in relation to risk of prostate cancer. *J Natl Cancer Inst* 87: 1767–1776, 1995.

40. Clinton SK, et al. Cis-trans lycopene isomers, carotenoids, and retinol in the human prostate. *Cancer Epidemiol Biomarkers Prevent* 5: 823–833, 1996.

41. Cohen M and Bhagavan HN. Ascorbic acid and gastrointestinal cancer. *J Am Coll Nutr* 14(6): 565–578, 1995.

42. Ocke M, Kromhout D, Menotti A, et al. Average intake of antioxidant (pro) vitamins and subsequent cancer mortality in the 16 cohorts of the Seven Countries study. *Int J Cancer* 61(4): 480–484, 1995.

43. Kromhout D and Bueno-de-Mesquita HB. Antioxidant vitamins and stomach cancer: the role of ecologic studies. *Cancer Lett* 114: 333–334, 1997.

44. Shibata A, et al. Intake of vegetables, fruits, beta-carotene, vitamin C and vitamin supplements and cancer incidence among the elderly: a prospective study. *Br J Cancer* 66(4): 673–679, 1992.

45. Cohen M and Bhagavan HN., 1995.

46. Esteve J, et al., 1996.

47. Flagg EW, Coates RJ, and Greenberg RS., 1995.

48. Block G. Epidemiologic evidence regarding vitamin C and cancer. *Am J Clin Nutr* 54: 1310S–1314S, 1991.

49. Daviglus ML, et al. Dietary beta-carotene, vitamin C, and risk of prostate cancer: results from the Western Electric study. *Epidemiology* 7(5): 472–477, 1996.

50. Bruemmer B, et al. Nutrient intake in relation to bladder cancer among middle-aged men and women. *Am J Epidemiol* 144(5): 485–495, 1996.

51. Otoole P and Lombard M. Vitamin C and gastric cancer: supplements for some or fruit for all. *Gut* 39(3): 345–347, 1996.

52. Greenberg ER, Baron JA, Tosteson TD, et al. A clinical trial of antioxidant vitamins to prevent colorectal adenoma. *N Engl J Med* 331: 141–147, 1994.

53. Kushi L, Fee R, Sellers T, et al. Intake of vitamins A, C, and E and postmenopausal breast cancer: the Iowa Women's Health Study. *Am J Epidemiol* 144(2): 165–174, 1996.

54. Hunter DJ, Manson JE, Colditz GA, et al. A prospective study of the intake of vitamins C, E, and A and the risk of breast cancer. *N Engl J Med* 329(4): 234–240, 1993.

55. Katiyar SK and Mukhtar H. Tea antioxidants in cancer chemoprevention. *J Cell Biochem* (Suppl.) 27: 59–67, 1997.

56. Wang ZY, et al. Inhibitory effects of black tea, green tea, decaffeinated black tea, and decaffeinated green tea on ultraviolet B light-induced skin carcinogenesis in 7,12-dimethylbenz[a]anthracene-initiated SKH-1 mice. *Cancer Res* 54(13): 3428–3435, 1994.

57. McCord H. More good news in tea leaves. *Prevention* 47(3): 51, 1995.

58. Yang CS and Wang ZY. Tea and cancer. *J Natl Cancer Inst* 85(13): 1038–1049, 1993.

59. Imai K, et al. Cancer-preventive effects of drinking green tea among a Japanese population. *Prev Med* 26(6): 769–775, 1997.

60. Ji BT, et al. Green tea consumption and the risk of pancreatic and colorectal cancers. *Int J Cancer* 70(3): 255–258, 1997.

61. Yu GP, et al. Green-tea consumption and risk of stomach cancer: A population-based case-control study in Shanghai, China. *Cancer Causes Control* 6(6): 532–538, 1995.

62. Stich HF. Teas and tea components as inhibitors of carcinogen formation in model systems and man. *Prev Med* 21: 377–384, 1992.

63. Komori A, et al. Anticarcinogenic activity of green tea polyphenols. *Jpn J Clin Oncol* 23(3): 186–190, 1993.

64. Messina MJ, et al. Soy intake and cancer risks: a review of the in vitro and in vivo data. *Nutr Cancer* 21: 113–131, 1994.

65. Adlercreutz H and Mazur W. Phyto-oestrogens and western diseases. *Ann Med* 29: 95–120, 1997.

66. Stoll BA. Eating to beat breast cancer: potential role for soy supplements. *Ann Oncol* 8: 223–225, 1997.

67. Day NE. Phyto-estrogens and hormonally dependent cancers. *Pathol Biol* 42(10): 1090, 1994.

68. Day NE, 1994.

69. Adlercreutz H and Mazur W, 1997.

70. Butterworth CE Jr. Effect of folate on cervical cancer: synergism among risk factors. *Ann NY Acad Sci* 669: 293–299, 1992.

71. Kim Y-I, Mason JB, et al. Folate, epithelial dysplasia and colon cancer. *Proc Assoc Am Physicians* 107: 218–227, 1995.

72. Tseng M, et al. Micronutrients and the risk of colorectal adenomas. *Am J Epidemiol* 144(11): 1005–1014, 1996.

73. Heimberger DC. Localized deficiencies of folic acid in aerodigestive tissues. *Ann N Y Acad Sci* 669: 87–96, 1992.

74. Heimberger DC, 1992.

75. Martinez ME, et al. Calcium, vitamin D, and the occurrence of colorectal cancer among women. *J Natl Cancer Inst* 88(19): 1375–1382, 1996.

76. Kearney J, et al. Calcium, vitamin D, and dairy foods and the occurrence of colon cancer in men. *Am J Epidemiol* 143(9): 907–917, 1996.

77. Adlercreutz H and Mazur W, 1997.

78. Serraino M and Thompson LU. The effect of flaxseed supplementation on the initiation and promotional stages of mammary tumorigenesis. *Nutr Cancer* 17: 153–159, 1992.

79. Bougnoix P, et al. Alpha-linolenic acid content of adipose breast tissue: a host determinant of the risk of early metastasis in breast cancer. *Br J Cancer* 70: 330–334, 1994.

80. Jang M, Cai L, Udeani GO, et al. Cancer chemopreventive activity of resveratrol, a natural product derived from grapes. *Science* 275: 218–220, 1997.

81. Personal communication from a colleague at City of Hope Med Center in Duarte, CA.

82. Kearney J, et al., 1996.

Canker Sores

1. Das SK, et al. Deglycyrrhizinated liquorice in apthous ulcers. *J Assoc Physicians India* 37: 647, 1989.

Cardiomyopathy

1. Langsjoen H, Langsjoen P, Langsjoen P, et al. Usefulness of coenzyme Q_{10} in clinical cardiology: a long-term study. *Mol Aspects Med* 15(Suppl. PS): 165–175, 1994.

2. Langsjoen PH, et al. Response of patients in classes III and IV of cardiomyopathy to therapy in a blind and crossover trial with coenzyme Q_{10}. *Proc Natl Acad Sci* 82: 4240, 1985.

3. Pogessi L, Galanti G, Comeglio M, et al. Effect of coenzyme Q_{10} on left ventricular function in patients with dilative cardiomyopathy. *Curr Ther Res* 49: 878–886, 1991.

4. Langsjoen PH, et al. A six-year clinical study of therapy of cardiomyopathy with coenzyme Q_{10}. *Int J Tissue React* 12(3): 169–171, 1990.

5. Langsjoen PH, et al. 1985.

6. Permanetter B, et al. Ubiquinone (coenzyme Q_{10}) in the long-term treatment of idiopathic dilated cardiomyopathy. *Eur Heart J* 13: 1528–1533, 1991.

7. Winter S, Jue K, Prochazka J, et al. The role of L-carnitine in pediatric cardiomyopathy. *J Child Neurol* (Canada) 10(Suppl. 2): 2S45–2S51, 1995.

8. Pepine CJ. The therapeutic potential of carnitine in cardiovascular disorders. *Clin Ther* 13(1): 2–21, 1991.

9. Bertelli A, et al. Carnitine and coenzyme Q_{10}: biochemical properties and functions, synergism and complementary action. *Int J Tissue React* 15(Suppl.): 183–186, 1990.

Cataracts

1. Hankinson S, Stampfer M, Seddon J, et al. Nutrient intake and cataract extraction in women: a prospective study. *BMJ* 305: 335–339, 1992.

2. Gerster H. No contribution of ascorbic acid to renal calcium oxalate stones. *Ann Nutr Metab* 41(5): 269–282, 1997.

3. Tavani A, et al. Food and nutrient intake and risk of cataract. *Ann Epidemiol* 6: 41–46, 1996.

4. Carson C, Lee S, De Paola C, et al. Antioxidant intake and cataract in the Melbourne Visual Impairment Project. *Am J Epidemiol* 139(11): S18, 1994.

5. Robertson JM, et al. Vitamin E intake and risk of cataracts in humans. *Ann NY Acad Sci* 570: 372–382, 1989.

6. Rouhiainen P, Rouhiainen H, Salonen J, et al. Association between low plasma vitamin E concentration and progression of early cortical lens opacities. *Am J Epidemiol* 144(5): 496–500, 1996.

7. Vitale S, West S, Hallfrish H, et al. Plasma antioxidants and risk of cortical and nuclear cataract. *Epidemiology* 4: 195–203, 1993.

8. Vitale S, et al. Plasma vitamin C, E and beta-carotene levels and risk of cataract. *Invest Ophthalmol Vis Sci* 32: 723, 1991.

9. Ross WM, Creighton MO, and Trevithick JR. Radiation cataractogenesis induced by neutron or gamma irradiation in the rat lens is reduced by vitamin E. *Scanning Microsc* 4: 641–650, 1990.

10. Albanes D, Heinonen OP, Huttunen JK, et al. Effects of alpha-tocopherol and beta-carotene supplements on cancer incidence in the Alpha-Tocopherol Beta-Carotene Cancer Prevention Study. *Am J Clin Nutr* 62(Suppl.): 1427S–1430S, 1995.

11. Bellizzi MC, Franklin MF, Duthie GG, et al. Vitamin E and coronary heart disease: the European paradox. *Eur J Clin Nutr* 48: 822–831, 1994.

12. Mares-Perlman JA, Brady WE, Klein BE, et al. Diet and nuclear lens opacities. *Am J Epidemiol* 141(4): 322–334, 1995.

13. Hankinson S, Stampfer M, Seddon J, et al. 1992.

14. Carson C, Lee S, De Paola C, et al., 1994.

15. Vitale S, West S, Hallfrish H, et al., 1993.

16. Bravetti G. Preventive medical treatment of senile cataract with vitamin E and anthocyanosides: clinical evaluation. *Ann Ottalmol Clin Ocul* 115: 109, 1989.

Cervical Dysplasia

1. Butterworth CE Jr, Hatch KD, Gore H, et al. Improvement in cervical dysplasia associated with folic acid therapy in users of oral contraceptives. *Am J Clin Nutr* 35(1): 73–82, 1982.

2. Zarcone R, Bellini P, Carfora E, et al. Folic acid and cervix dysplasia. *Minerva Ginecol* 48: 397–400, 1996.

3. Childers JM, Chu J, Voigt LF, et al. Chemoprevention of cervical cancer with folic acid: a phase III Southwest Oncology Group Intergroup study. *Cancer Epidemiol Biomarkers Prev* 4(2): 155–159, 1995.

4. Butterworth CE Jr, Hatch KD, Soong SJ, et al. Oral folic acid supplementation for cervical dysplasia: a clinical intervention trial. *Am J Obstet Gynecol* 166(30): 803–809, 1992.

5. Orr J, et al. Nutritional status of patients with untreated cervical cancer I and II. *Am J Obstet Gynecol* 151: 625–635, 1985.

6. Romney SL, et al. Nutrient antioxidants in the pathogenesis and prevention of cervical dysplasia and cancer. *J Cell Biochem* 23: 96–103, 1995.

7. Butterworth CE Jr. Effect of folate on cervical cancer. Synergism among risk factors. *Ann NY Acad Sci* 669: 293–299, 1992.

Cholesterol

1. Mader FH. Treatment of hyperlipidaemia with garlic-powder tablets: evidence from the German Association of General Practitioners' multicentric placebo-controlled double-blind study. *Arzneimittelforschung* 40(10): 1111–1116, 1990.

2. Neil HA, et al. Garlic powder in the treatment of moderate hyperlipidaemia: a controlled trial and meta-analysis. *J R Coll Physicians Lond* 30(4): 329–334,1990.

3. Simons LA, et al. On the effect of garlic on plasma lipids and lipoproteins in mild hypercholesterolaemia. *Atherosclerosis* 13(2): 219–225, 1995.

4. Silagy CA, et al. A meta-analysis of the effect of garlic on blood pressure. *J Hypertens* 12(4): 463–468, 1994.

5. Warshafsky S, et al. Effect of garlic on total serum cholesterol: a meta-analysis. *Ann Intern Med* 119(Pt. 1): 599–605, 1993.

6. Steiner M, et al. A double-blind crossover study in moderately hypercholesterolemic men that compared the effect of aged garlic extract and placebo administration on blood lipids. *Am J Clin Nutr* 64(6): 866–870, 1996.

7. Santos OS de A, et al. Effects of garlic powder and garlic oil preparations on blood lipids, blood pressure and well being. *Br J Clin Res* 6: 91–100, 1995.

8. Breithaupt-Grogler K, et al. Protective effect of chronic garlic intake on the elastic properties of the aorta in the elderly. *Circulation* 96(7): 2649–2655, 1997.

9. Schulz V, et al. Rational phytotherapy. New York: Springer-Verlag, 1998.

10. Agarwal KC, et al. Therapeutic actions of garlic constituents. *Med Res Rev* 16(1): 111–124, 1996.

11. Legnani C, et al. Effects of dried garlic preparation on fibrinolysis and platelet aggregation in health subjects. *Arzneimittelforschung* 43: 119–121, 1993.

12. Chutani SK, et al. The effect of dried vs. raw garlic on fibrinolytic activity in man. *Atherosclerosis* 38: 417–421, 1981.

13. Kiesewetter H, et al. Effect of garlic on thrombocyte aggregation, microcirculation and other risk factors. *Int J Clin Pharmacol Ther Toxicol* 29: 151–155, 1991.

14. Reuter HD, et al. *Allium sativum* and *Allium ursinum:* chemistry, pharmacology and medical applications. *Econo Med Plant Res* 6: 56–108, 1994.

15. Popov I, et al. Antioxidant effects of aqueous garlic extract, 1st communication: direct detection using photochemoluminescence. *Arzneimittelforschung Drug Res* 44(1): 602–604, 1994.

16. Torok B, et al. Effectiveness of garlic on radical activity in radical generating systems. *Arzneimittelforschung Drug Res* 44(1): 608–611, 1994.

17. Sumiyoshi H, et al. Chronic toxicity test of garlic extracts in rats. *J Toxicol Sci* 9: 61–75, 1984.

18. Schulz V, et al., 1998.

19. Beck E, et al. *Allium sativum* in der Stufentherapie der Hyperlipidamie *Med Welt* 44: 516–520, 1993. As cited in Schulz V, et al. Rational phytotherapy. New York: Springer-Verlag, 1998.

20. Heber D, et al. Cholesterol-lowering effects of a proprietary Chinese red yeast rice dietary supplement. *FASEB J* 12(4): A206, 1998.

21. Chang M. Cholestin: health-care professional product guide. Simi Valley: Pharmanex, 1998: 1–6.

22. Crouse JR III. New developments in the use of niacin for treatment of hyperlipidemia: new considerations in the use of an old drug. *Coron Artery Dis* 7: 321–326, 1996.

23. Head KA. Inositol hexaniacinate: a safer alternative to niacin. *Alt Med Rev* 1: 176–184, 1996.

24. Glore SR, et al. Soluble fiber and serum lipids: a literature review. *J Am Diet Assoc* 94: 425–436, 1994.

25. Anderson JW, Johnstone BM, and Cook-Newell ME. Meta-analysis of the effects of soy protein intake on serum lipids. *N Engl J Med* 333: 276–282, 1995.

26. Agarwal RC, et al. Clinical trial of gugulipid: a new hyperlipidemic agent of plant origin in primary hyperlipidemia. *Indian J Med Res* 84: 626–634, 1986.

27. Nityanand, S, et al. Clinical trials with gugulipid. A new hypolipidaemic agent. *J Assoc Physicians India* 37(5): 323–328, 1989.

28. Singh RB, et al. Hypolipidemic and antioxidant effects of Commiphora mukul as an adjunct to dietary therapy in patients with hypercholesterolemia. *Cardiovasc Drug Ther* 8(4): 659–664, 1994.

29. Gaddi A, et al. Controlled evaluation of pantethine, a natural hypolipidemic compound, in patients with different forms of hyperlipoproteinemia. *Atherosclerosis* 50(1): 73–83, 1984.

30. Rubba R, Postiglione A, DeSimone B, et al. Comparative evaluation of the lipid-lowering effects of fenofibrate and pantethine in type II hyperlipoproteinemia. *Curr Ther Res Clin Exp* 38: 719–727, 1985.

31. Angelico M, et al. Improvement in serum lipid profile in hyperlipoproteinaemic patients after treatment with pantethine: a crossover, double-blind trial versus placebo. *Curr Ther Res* 33: 1091, 1983.

32. Davini P, et al. Controlled study on L-carnitine therapeutic efficacy in post-infarction. *Drugs Exp Clin Res* 18(8): 355–365, 1992.

33. Vecchio F, Zanchin G, Maggioni F, et al. Mesoglycan in treatment of patients with cerebral ischemia: effects on hemorrheologic and hematochemical parameters. *Acta Neurol* (Napoli) 15(6): 449–456, 1993.

34. Saba P, Galeone F, Giuntoli F, et al. Hypolipidemic effect of mesoglycan in hyperlipidemic patients. *Curr Ther Res* 40: 761–768, 1986.

35. Postiglione A, De Simone B, Rubba P, et al. Effect of oral mesoglycan on plasma lipoprotein concentration and on lipoprotein lipase activity in primary hyperlipidemia. *Pharmacol Res Commun* 16(1): 1–8, 1984.

36. Mertz W. Chromium in human nutrition: a review. *J Nutr* 123: 626–633, 1993.

37. Bell L, et al. Cholesterol-lowering effects of calcium carbonate in patients with mild to moderate hypercholesterolemia. *Arch Intern Med* 152: 2441–2444, 1992.

38. Schwarz B, Bischof H, Kunze M. Coffee, tea and lifestyle. *Prev Med* 23: 377–384, 1994.

Colds and Flus

1. Dorn M. Milderung grippaler Effekte durch ein pflanzliches Immunstimulans. *Natur und Ganzheitsmedizin*. As cited in Schulz V, et al. Rational phytotherapy. New York: Springer-Verlag, 1998: 277.

2. Braunig B, et al. *Echinacea purpurea* root for strengthening the immune response in flu-like infections. *Z Phytother* 13: 7–13, 1992.

3. Dorn M, et al. Placebo-controlled double-blind study of *Echinacea pallidae radix* in upper respiratory tract infections. *Complement Ther Med* 3: 40–42, 1997.

4. Hoheisel O, et al. Echinagard treatment shortens the course of the common cold: a double-blind placebo-controlled clinical trial. *Eur J of Clin Res* 9: 261–268, 1997.

5. Melchart MD, et al. Immunomodulation with echinacea—A sytematic review of controlled clinical trials. *Phytomedicine* 1: 245–254, 1994.

6. Melchart, MD, et al. Echinacea root extracts for the prevention of upper respiratory tract infections: a double-blind, placebo-controlled randomized trial. *Arch Fam Med* 7: 541–545, 1998.

7. Schoenberger D. The influence of immune-stimulating effects of pressed juice from *Echinacea purpurea* on the course and severity of colds. *Forum Immunol* 8: 2–12, 1992.

8. Bauer R, et al. Echinacea species as potential immunostimulatory drugs. *Econ Med Plant Res* 5: 253–321, 1991.

9. Wagner V, et al. Immunostimulating polysaccharides (heteroglycans) of higher plants. *Arzneimittelforschung* 35: 1069–1075, 1985.

10. Stimpel M, et al. Macrophage activation and induction of macrophage cytotoxicity by purified polysaccharide fractions from the plant *Echinacea purpurea*. *Infect Immun* 46: 845–849, 1984.

11. Luettig B, et al. Macrophage activation by the polysaccharide arabinogalactan isolated from plant cell cultures of *Echinacea purpurea*. *J Natl Cancer Inst* 81: 669–675, 1989.

12. Mose J. Effect of echinacin on phagocytosis and natural killer cells. *Med Welt* 34: 1463–1467, 1983.

13. Vomel V. Influence of a non-specific immune stimulant on phagocytosis of erythrocytes and ink by the reticuloendothelial system of isolated perfused rat livers of different ages. *Arzneimittelforschung* 34: 691–695, 1984.

14. Hobbs C. The echinacea handbook. Portland, OR: Eclectic Medical Publications, 1989.

15. Schulz V, et al. Rational phytotherapy. New York: Springer-Verlag, 1998: 278.

16. Bergner P. Goldenseal and the common cold: the antibiotic myth. *Med Herbalism* 8(4): 1–10, 1997.

17. Schulz V, et al., 1998.

18. Mengs U, et al. Toxicity of *Echinacea purpurea* acute, subacute and genotoxicity studies. *Arzneimittelforschung Drug Res* 41(11): 1076–1081, 1991.

19. Parnham MJ. Benefit-risk assessment of the squeezed sap of the purple coneflower *(Echinacea purpurea)* for long-term oral immunostimulation. *Phytomedicine* 3(1): 99–102, 1996.

20. Parnham MJ, 1996.

21. Melchior J, et al. Controlled clinical study of standardized *Andrographis paniculata* extract in common cold: a pilot trial. *Phytomedicine* 34: 314–318, 1996–1997.

22. Hancke J, et al. A double-blind study with a new monodrug Kan Jang: decrease of symptoms and improvements in the recovery from common colds. *Phytother Res* 9: 559–562, 1995.

23. Thamlikitkul V, et al. Efficacy of *Andrographis paniculata* (Nees) for pharyngotonsillitis in adults. *J Med Assoc Thai* 74(10): 437–442, 1991.

24. Hancke J, et al., 1996–1997.

25. Akbarsha MA, et al. Antifertility effect of *Andrographis paniculata* (Nees) in male albino rat. *Indian J Exp Biol* 28(5): 421–426, 1990.

26. Burgos RA, et al. Testicular toxicity assessment of *Andrographis paniculata* dried extract in rats. *J Ethnopharmacol* 58(3): 219–224, 1997.

27. Zoha MS, et al. Antifertility effect of *Andrographis paniculata* in mice. *Bangladesh Med Res Counc Bull* 15(1): 34–37, 1989.

28. Chandra RK. Trace element regulation of immunity and infection. *J Am Coll Nutr* 4(1): 5–16, 1985.

29. Fraker PJ, et al. interrelationships between zinc and immune function. *Fed Proc* 45(5): 1474–1479, 1986.

30. Werbach M. Nutritional influences on illness. CD-ROM. Tarzana, CA: Third Line Press, 1998: 630.

31. Girodon F, Lombard M, Galan P, et al. Effect of micronutrient supplementation on infection in institutionalized elderly subjects: a controlled trial. *Ann Nutr Metab* 41(2): 98–107, 1997.

32. Mossad SB, et al. Zinc gluconate lozenges for treating the common cold: a randomized, double-blind placebo-controlled study. *Ann Intern Med* 125: 142–144, 1996.

33. Macknin ML, et al. Zinc gluconate lozenges for treating the common cold in children: a randomized controlled trial. *JAMA* 279(24): 1962–1967, 1998.

34. Marshall S. Zinc gluconate and the common cold: review of randomized controlled trials. *Can Fam Physician* 44: 1037–1042, 1998.

35. Eby GA. Zinc ion availability—the determinant of efficacy in zinc lozenge treatment of common colds. *Antimicrob Chemother* 40(4): 483–493, 1997.

36. Macknin ML, et al., 1998.

37. Hemilä H. Vitamin C and the common cold. *Br J Nutr* 67: 3–16, 1992.

38. Hemilä H. Does vitamin C alleviate symptoms of the common cold?—a review of current evidence. *Scand J Infect Dis* 26: 1–6, 1994.

39. Peters EM, Goetzsche JM, Grobbelaar B, et al. Vitamin C supplementation reduces the incidence of postrace symptoms of upper-respiratory-tract infection in ultramarathon runners. *Am J Clin Nutr* 57(2): 170–174, 1993.

40. Hemilä H. Vitamin C and common cold incidence: a review of studies with subjects under heavy physical stress. *Int J Sports Med* 17(5): 379–383, 1996.

41. Hemilä H. Vitamin C intake and susceptibility to the common cold. *Br J Nutr* 77: 1–14, 1997.

42. Scaglione F, et al. Efficacy and safety of the standardised ginseng extract G115 for potentiating vaccination against the influenza syndrome and protection against the common cold. *Drugs Exp Clin Res* 22(2): 65–72, 1996.

43. Ploss E. *Panax ginseng.* C. A. Meyer. Scientific report. Cologne: Kooperation Phytopharmaka, 1998.

44. Lawrence Review of Natural Products. Ginseng monograph, St. Louis, Missouri: Facts and Comparisons Division, J.B. Lipincott Company, March, 1990.

45. Tyler V. Herbs of choice. New York: Pharmaceutical Production Press, 1994.

46. Tyler V., 1994.

47. Schulz V, et al. 1998: 271, 273.

48. Meydani SM, et al. Vitamin E supplementation and in vivo immune response in healthy elderly subjects: a randomized controlled trial. *JAMA* 277: 1380–1386, 1997.

49. Zakay-Rones Z, et al. Inhibition of several strains of influenza virus and reduction of symptoms by an elderberry extract (*Sambucus nigra* L.) during an outbreak of influenza B Panama. *J Altern Complement Med* 1(4): 361–369, 1995.

Congestive Heart Failure

1. Hofman-Bang C, et al. Coenzyme Q_{10} as an adjunctive treatment of congestive heart failure. *J Am Coll Cardiol* 19: 216A, 1992.

2. Morisco C, et al. Effect of coenzyme Q_{10} therapy in patients with congestive heart failure: a long-term multicenter randomized study. *Clin Invest* 71(Suppl. 8): S134–S136, 1993.

3. Lampetico M, et al. Italian multicenter study on the efficacy and safety of coenzyme Q_{10} as adjuvant therapy in heart failure. *Clin Invest* 71(Suppl. 8): S129–S133, 1993.

4. Popping S, et al. Effect of a hawthorn extract on contraction and energy turnover of isolated rat cardiomyocytes. *Arzneimittelforschung Drug Res* 45: 1157–1161, 1995.

5. Joseph G. Pharmacologic action profile of crataegus extract in comparison to epinephrine, amirinone, milrinone and digoxin in the isolated perfused guinea pig heart. *Arzneimittelforschung* 45(12): 1261–1265, 1995.

6. Schulz V, et al., Rational phytotherapy. New York: Springer-Verlag, 1998.

7. Schulz V, et al., 1998: 91–94.

8. Schulz V, et al., 1998: 90–98.

9. Schulz V, et al., 1998: 95.

10. Azuma J, et al. Therapy of congestive heart failure with orally administered taurine. *Clin Ther* 5(4): 398–408, 1983.

11. Azuma J, et al. Double-blind randomized crossover trial of taurine in congestive heart failure. *Curr Ther Res* 34(4): 543–557, 1983.

12. Caponnetto S, et al. Efficacy of L-propionylcarnitine treatment in patients with left ventricular dysfunction. *Eur Heart J* 15(9): 1267–1273, 1994.

13. Mancini M, et al. Controlled study on the therapeutic efficacy of propionyl-L-carnitine in patients with congestive heart failure. *Arzneimittelforschung* 42: 1101–1104, 1992.

14. Cacciatore L, et al. The therapeutic effect of L-carnitine in patients with exercise-induced stable angina: A controlled study. *Drugs Exp Clin Res* 17: 225–235, 1991.

15. Pucciarelli G, et al. The clinical and hemodynamic effects of propionyl-L-carnitine in patients with congestive heart failure. *Clin Ther* 141: 379–384, 1992.

Cyclic Mastalgia

1. Horrobin DF, et al. Abnormalities in plasma essential fatty acid levels in women with premenstrual syndrome and with nonmalignant breast disease. *J Nutr Med* 2: 259–264, 1991.

2. Pye JK, et al. Clinical experience of drug treatment for mastalgia. *Lancet* ii: 373–377, 1985.

3. Pashby NL, et al. A clinical trial of evening primrose oil in mastalgia. *Br J Surg* 68: 801–824, 1981.

4. Mansel RE, et al. Effect and tolerability of n-6 essential fatty acid supplementation in patients with recurrent breast cysts—a randomized double-blind placebo-controlled trial. *J Nutr Med* 1: 195–200, 1990.

5. Mansel RE, et al. A randomized trial of dietary intervention with essential fatty acids in patients with categorized cysts. *Ann NY Acad Sci* 586: 288–294, 1990.

6. Tamborini A, et al. Value of standardized *Ginkgo biloba* extract in the management of congestive symptoms of premenstrual syndrome. *Rev Fr Gynecol Obstet* 88(7–9): 447–457, 1993.

7. De Feudis FV. *Ginkgo biloba* extract: Pharmacological activity and clinical applications. Paris: Elsevier, 1991: 143–146.

8. Kleijnen J and Knipschild P. *Ginkgo biloba* for cerebral insufficiency. *Br J Clin Pharamcol* 34: 352–358, 1992.

9. De Feudis FV., 1991.

10. Dittmar FW, et al. Premenstrual syndrome: treatment with a phytopharmaceutical. *Therapie Gynakol* 5: 60–68, 1992.

11. Peteres-Welte C, et al. Menstrual abnormalities and PMS: *Vitex agnus-castus*. *Therapie Gynakol* 7: 49–52, 1994.

12. Coeugniet E, et al. Premenstrual syndrome (PMS) and its treatment. *Arztezeitschr Naturheilverf* 27: 619–622, 1986.

Depression

1. Laakman G, et al. St. John's wort in mild to moderate depression: the relevance of hyperforin for the clinical efficacy. *Pharmacopsychiatry* 31 (Suppl.): 54–59, 1998.

2. Linde K, et al. St. John's wort for depression—an overview and meta-analysis of randomized clinical trials. *BMJ* 313: 253–258, 1996.

3. Ernst E. St. John's wort, an antidepressant? A systematic, criteria-based review. *Phytomedicine* 2(1): 67–71, 1995.

4. Suzuki O, et al. Inhibition of monoamine oxidase by hypericin. *Planta Medica* 50: 2722–2724, 1984.

5. Bladt S, et al. Inhibition of MAO by fractions and constituents of hypericum extract. *J Geriatr Psychiatry Neurol* 7(Suppl. 1): S57–S59, 1994.

6. Thiede B, et al. Inhibition of MAO and COMT by hypericum extracts and hypericin. *J Geriatr Psychiatry Neurol* 7(Suppl. 1): 54–56, 1994.

7. Muller WEG, et al. Effects of hypericum extract on the expression of serotonin receptors. *J Geriatr Psychiatry Neurol* 7(Suppl. 1): S63–S64, 1994.

8. Muller WE, et al. Hypericum extract (LI160) as an herbal antidepressant. *Pharmacopsychiatry* 30(Suppl. 2): 71–134, 1997.

9. Laakman G, et al., 1998.

10. Woelk H, et al. Benefits and risks of the hypericum extract LI 160: drug monitoring study with 3,250 patients. *J Geriatr Psychiatry Neurol* 7(Suppl 1): S34–S38, 1994.

11. Smet P and Nolen W. St. John's wort as an antidepressant. *BMJ* 3: 241–242, 1996.

12. Schulz V, et al. Rational phytotherapy. New York: Springer-Verlag, 1998: 56.

13. Seigers CP, et al. Phototoxicity caused by hypericum. *Nervenhielkunde* 12: 320–322, 1993.

14. Brockmoller J, et al. Hypericin and pseudohypericin: pharmacokinetics and effects on photosensitivity in humans. *Pharmacopsychiatry* 30(Suppl. 2): 94–101, 1997.

15. Suzuki O, et al., 1984.

16. Bladt S, et al., 1994.

17. Thiede B, et al., 1994.

18. Baker RK, et al. Inhibition of human DNA topoisomerase IIalpha by the naphthodianthrone, hypericin. *Proc Am Assoc Cancer Res* 39: 422, 1998.

19. Nebel A, et al. Potential metabolic interaction between theophylline and St. John's wort. Submitted to *Ann Pharmacother*, 1998.

20. Baker RK, et al. Catalytic inhibition of human DNA topoisomerase IIalpha by hypericin, a naphthodianthone from St. John's wort *(Hypericum perforatum).* Manuscript in preparation.

21. Heller B. Pharmacological and clinical effects of D-phenylalanine in depression and Parkinson's disease. As cited in Mosnaim and Wolf, eds. Noncatecholic phenylethylamines, Part 1. New York: Marcel Dekker, 1978: 397–417.

22. Beckmann H, et al. DL-phenylalanine versus imipramine: a double-blind controlled study. *Arch Psychiat Nervenkr* 227: 49–58, 1979.

23. Beckmann H. Phenylalanine in affective disorders. *Adv Biol Psychiatry* 10: 137–147, 1983.

24. Byerly WF, et al. 5-hydroxytryptophan: a review of its antidepressant efficacy and adverse effects. *J Clin Psychopharmacol* 7: 127–137, 1987.

25. Poldinger W, et al. A functional-dimensional approach to depression: serotonin deficiency as a target syndrome in a comparison of 5-hydroxytryptophan and fluvoxamine. *Psychopathology* 24: 53–81, 1991.

26. Eckmann F. Cerebral insufficiency treatment with *Ginkgo-biloba* extract: time of onset of effect in a double-blind study with 60 inpatients. *Fortschr Med* 108: 557–560, 1990.

27. Schubert H, et al. Depressive episode primarily unresponsive to therapy in elderly patients: efficacy of *Ginkgo-biloba* (EGb 761) in combination with antidepressants. *Geriatr Forsch* 3: 45–53, 1993.

28. Huguet F, et al. Decreased cerebral 5-HT receptors during aging: reversal by *Ginkgo-biloba* extract (EGb 761). *J Pharm Pharmacol* 46: 316–318, 1994.

29. Schulz V, et al. 1998: 41.

30. De Feudis FV. *Ginkgo biloba* extract (EGb 761): Pharmacological activity and clinical applications. Paris: Elsevier, 1991: 143–146.

31. Cenacchi T, et al. Cognitive decline in the elderly: a double-blind, placebo-controlled multicenter study on efficacy of phosphatidylserine administration. *Aging* 5: 123–133, 1993.

32. Benjamen J, et al. Inositol treatment in psychiatry. *Psychopharmacol Bull* 31(1): 167–175, 1995.

33. Bell I, et al. Complex vitamin patterns in geriatric and young adult inpatients with major depression. *J Am Geriatr Soc* 39: 252–257, 1991.

34. Zucker DK et al. B_{12} deficiency and psychiatric disorders: case report and literature review. *Biol Psychiatry* 16: 197–205, 1981.

35. Alpert JE and Fava M. Nutrition and depression: the role of folate. *Nutr Rev* 55(5): 145–149, 1997.

Diabetes

1. Anderson RA, et al. Elevated intakes of supplemental chromium improve glucose and insulin variables in individuals with type II diabetes. *Diabetes* 46(11): 1786–1791, 1997.

2. Ravina A, et al. Chromium in the treatment of clinical diabetes mellitus. *Harefuah* 125(5–6): 142–145, 1993.

3. Rabinowitz MB, et al. Effect of chromium and yeast supplements on carbohydrate and lipid metabolism in diabetic men. *Diabetes Care* 6: 319–327, 1983.

4. Certulli J, et al. Chromium picolinate toxicity. *Ann Pharmacother* 32: 428–431, 1998.

5. Wasser WG, et al. Chronic renal failure after ingestion of over-the-counter chromium picolinate. *Ann Intern Med* 126(5): 410, 1997.

6. Sharma RD, Sarkar A, Hazra DK, et al. Use of fenugreek seed powder in the management of non-insulin-dependent diabetes mellitus. *Nutr Res* 16: 1331–1339, 1996.

7. Madar Z, et al. Glucose-lowering effect of fenugreek in non-insulin-dependent diabetics. *Eur J Clin Nutr* 42: 51–54, 1988.

8. Sharma RD, Raghuram TC, and Rao NS. Effect of fenugreek seeds on blood glucose and serum lipids in type I diabetes. *Eur J Clin Nutr* 44: 301–306, 1990.

9. Leung A, et al. Encyclopedia of common natural ingredients in food, drugs, and cosmetics. New York: John Wiley and Sons, 1996: 243–244.

10. Baskaran K, et al. Antidiabetic effect of a leaf extract from *Gymnema sylvestre* in non-insulin-dependent diabetes mellitus patients. *J Ethnopharmacol* 30: 295–305, 1990.

11. Shanmugasundaram ERB, et al. Use of *Gymnema sylvestre* leaf extract in the control of blood glucose in insulin-dependent diabetes mellitus. *J Ethnopharmacol* 30: 281–294, 1990.

12. Authors not noted. Flexible dose open trial of Vijayasar in cases of newly-diagnosed non-insulin-dependent diabetes mellitus. Indian Council of Medical Research (ICMR), Collaborating Centres, New Delhi. *Indian J Med Res* 108: 24–29, 1998.

13. Sotaneimi EA, et al. Ginseng therapy in non-insulin-dependent diabetic patients. *Diabetes Care* 18(10): 1373–1375, 1995.

14. Yaniv Z, Dafni A, Friedman J, et al. Plants used for the treatment of diabetes in Israel. *J Ethnopharmacol* 19(2): 145–151, 1987.

15. Teixeira CC, et al. The effect of *Syzygium cumini* (L.) skeels on post-prandial blood glucose levels in non-diabetic rats and rats with streptozotocin-induced diabetes mellitus. *J Ethnopharmacol* 56: 209–213, 1997.

16. Bever BO and Zahnd GR. Plants with oral hypoglycemic action. *Q J Crude Drug Res* 17: 139–196, 1979.

17. Mathew PT and Augusti KT. Hypoglycaemic effects of onion, *Allium cepa* Linn. on diabetes mellitus—a preliminary report. *Indian J Physiol Pharmacol* 19: 213–217, 1975.

18. Manickam M, Ramanathan M, Jahromi MA, et al. Antihyperglycemic activity of phenolics from *Pterocarpus marsupium*. *J Nat Prod* 60: 609–610, 1997.

19. Ahmad F, Khalid P, Khan MM, et al. Insulin like activity in (-) epicatechin. *Acta Diabetol Lat* 26: 291–300, 1989.

20. Stern E. Successful use of *Atriplex halimus* in the treatment of type 2 diabetic patients: a preliminary study. Zamenhoff Medical Center, Tel Aviv, 1989.

21. Earon G, Stern E, and Lavosky H. Successful use of *Atriplex hamilus* in the treatment of type 2 diabetic patients. Controlled clinical research report on the subject of Atriplex. Unpublished study conducted at the Hebrew University, Jerusalem, 1989.

22. Khan AK, Akhtar S, and Mahtab H. Treatment of diabetes mellitus with *Coccinia indica*. *BMJ* 280: 1044, 1980.

23. Welihinda J, et al. Effect of *Momordica charantia* on the glucose tolerance in maturity onset diabetes. *J Ethnopharmacol* 17: 277–282, 1986.

24. Akhtar MS. Trial of *Momordica charantia* Linn (Karela) powder in patients with maturity-onset diabetes. *J Pak Med Assoc* 32: 106–107, 1982.

25. Leatherdale BA, Panesar RK, Singh G, et al. Improvement of glucose tolerance due to *Momordica charantia* (Karela). *BMJ* (Clin Res Ed) 282: 1823–1824, 1981.

26. Cignarella A, et al. Novel lipid-lowering properties of *Vaccinium myrtillus* L. leaves, a traditional antidiabetic treatment, in several models of rat dyslipidaemia: a comparison with ciprofibrate. *Thromb Res* 84: 311–322, 1996.

27. Paolisso G, D'Amore A, Galzerano D, et al. Daily vitamin E supplements improve metabolic control but not insulin secretion in elderly non-insulin-dependent diabetic patients. *Diabetes Care* 16: 1433–1437, 1993.

28. Paolisso G, D'Amore A, Giugliano D, et al. Pharmacologic doses of vitamin E improve insulin action in healthy subjects and non-insulin-dependent diabetic patients. *Am J Clin Nutr* 57: 650–656, 1993.

29. Kagan VE, et al. Dihydrolipoic acid—A universal antioxidant both in the membrane in the aqueous phase. *Biochem Pharmacol* 44: 1637–1649, 1992.

30. Packer L, Witt EH, and Tritschler HJ. Alpha-lipoic acid as a biological antioxidant. *Free Radical Biol Med* 19: 227–250, 1995.

31. Ziegler D, et al. Alpha-lipoic acid in the treatment of diabetic peripheral and cardiac autonomic neuropathy. *Diabetes* 46(Suppl. 2): S62–S66, 1997.

32. Kahler W, et al. Diabetes mellitus—A free radical–associated disease: results of adjuvant antioxidant supplementation. *Gesamte Inn Med* 48: 223–232, 1993.

33. Ziegler D, et al., 1997.

34. Stevens EJ, et al. Essential fatty acid treatment prevents nerve ischaemia and associated conduction anomalies in rats with experimental diabetes mellitus. *Diabetologia* 36(5): 397–401, 1993.

35. Reichert RG. Evening primrose oil and diabetic neuropathy. *Q Rev Natl Med*: 141–145, 1995.

36. Keen H, et al. Treatment of diabetic neuropathy with gamma-linolenic acid: the gamma-linolenic acid multicenter trial group. *Diabetes Care* 16(1): 8–15, 1993.

37. Horrobin DF. The use of gamma-linolenic acid in diabetic neuropathy. *Agents Actions* (Suppl.) 37: 120–144, 1992.

38. Horrobin DF. Nutritional and medical importance of gamma-linolenic acid. *Prog Lipid Res* 31: 163–194, 1992.

39. Horrobin DF, et al. Gamma-linolenic acid: an intermediate in essential fatty acid metabolism with potential as an ethical pharmaceutical and as a food. *Rev Contemp Pharmacother* 1: 1–45, 1990.

40. Horrobin DF. Essential fatty acids in the management of impaired nerve function in diabetes. *Diabetes* 46(Suppl. 2): S90–S93, 1997.

41. Vaddadi KS. The use of gamma-linolenic acid and linoleic acid to differentiate between temporal lobe epilepsy and schizophrenia. *Prostaglandins Med* 6: 375–379, 1981.

42. Horrobin DF. The regulation of prostaglandin biosynthesis by the manipulation of essential fatty acid metabolism. *Rev Pure Appl Pharmacol* 4: 339–383, 1983.

43. Bravetti G. Preventive medical treatment of senile cataract with vitamin E and anthocyanosides: clinical evaluation. *Ann Ottalmol Clin Ocul* 115: 109, 1989.

44. Scharrer A, et al. Anthocyanosides in the treatment of retinopathies. *Klin Monatsbl Augenheilkd* 178: 386–389, 1981.

45. Carson C, Lee S, De Paola C, et al. Antioxidant intake and cataract in the Melbourne Visual Impairment Project. *Am J Epidemiol* 139(11): S18, 1994.

46. Hankinson S, Stampfer M, Seddon J, et al. Nutrient intake and cataract extraction in women: a prospective study. *BMJ* 305: 335–339, 1992.

47. Will JC, et al. Does diabetes mellitus increase the requirement for vitamin C? *Nutr Rev* 54: 193–202, 1996.

48. Elamin A and Tuvemo T. Magnesium and insulin-dependent diabetes mellitus. *Diabetes Res Clin Pract* 10: 203–209, 1990.

49. Tosiello L. Hypomagnesemia and diabetes mellitus. *Arch Intern Med* 156: 1143–1148, 1996.

50. Schmidt LE, Arfken CL, and Heins JM. Evaluation of nutrient intake in subjects with non-insulin-dependent diabetes mellitus. *J Am Diet Assoc* 94(7): 773–774, 1994.

51. Blostein-Fujii A, DeSilvestro RA, Frid D, et al. Short-term zinc supplementation in women with non-insulin-dependent diabetes mellitus: effects on plasma 5'-nucleotidase activities, insulin-like growth factor I concentrations, and lipoprotein oxidation rates in vitro. *Am J Clin Nutr* 66: 639–642, 1997.

52. Sjogren A, Floren CH, and Nilsson A. Magnesium, potassium and zinc deficiency in subjects with type II diabetes mellitus. *Acta Med Scand* 224: 461–466, 1988.

53. Cunningham J. Reduced mononuclear leukocyte ascorbic acid content in adults with insulin-dependent diabetes mellitus consuming adequate dietary vitamin C. *Metabolism* 40: 146–149, 1991.

54. Sinclair AJ, et al. Low plasma ascorbate levels in patients with type 2 diabetes mellitus consuming adequate dietary vitamin C. *Diabet Med* 11: 893–898, 1994.

55. Will JC, et al., 1996.

56. Singh RB, et al. Dietary intake and plasma levels of antioxidant vitamins in health and disease: a hospital-based case-control study. *J Nutr Environ Med* 5: 235–242, 1995.

57. Basu TK, et al. Serum vitamin A and retinol-binding protein in patients with insulin-dependent diabetes mellitus. *Am J Clin Nutr* 50: 329–331, 1989.

58. Wako Y, et al. Vitamin A transport in plasma of diabetic patients. *Tohoku J Exp Med* 149: 133–143, 1986.

59. Franconi F, Bennardini F, Mattana A, et al. Plasma and platelet taurine are reduced in subjects with insulin-dependent diabetes mellitus: effects of taurine supplementation. *Am J Clin Nutr* 61: 1115–1119, 1995.

Dysmenorrhea

1. Harel Z, Biro FM, Kottenhahn RK, et al. Supplementation with omega-3 polyunsaturated fatty acids in the management of dysmenorrhea in adolescents. *Am J Obstet Gynecol* 174(4): 1335–1338, 1996.

2. Harel Z, Biro FM, Kottenhahn RK, et al., 1996.

3. Fontana-Klaiber H, Hogg B. Therapeutic effects of magnesium in dysmenorrhea. *Schweiz Rundsch Med Prax* 79(16): 491–494, 1990.

4. Seifert B, et al. Magnesium—A new therapeutic alternative in primary dysmenorrhea. *Zentralbl Gynakol* 111(11): 755–760, 1989.

Eczema

1. Morse PF, et al. Meta-analysis of placebo-controlled studies of the efficacy of Epogam in the treatment of atopic eczema: relationship between plasma essential fatty acid changes and clinical response. *Br J Dermatol* 121(1): 75–90, 1989.

2. Berth-Jones J and Graham-Brown RAC. Placebo-controlled trial of essential fatty acid supplementation in atopic dermatitis. *Lancet* 341: 1557–1560, 1993.

3. Hederos CA, et al. Epogam evening primrose oil treatment in atopic dermatitis and asthma. *Arch Dis Child* 75(6): 494–497, 1996.

4. Whitaker DK, et al. Evening primrose oil (Epogam) in the treatment of chronic hand dermatitis: disappointing therapeutic results. *Dermatology* 193: 115–120, 1996.

5. Bamford JT, et al. Atopic eczema unresponsive to evening primrose oil (linoleic and gamma-linolenic acids). *J Am Acad Dermatol* 13: 959–965, 1985.

6. Horrobin DF and Stewart C. Evening primrose oil in atopic eczema (letter). *Lancet* i: 864–865, 1990.

7. Wright S. Essential fatty acids in clinical dermatology. *J Nutr Med* 1: 301–313, 1990.

8. Biagi PL, et al. The effect of gamma-linolenic acid on clinical status, red cell fatty acid composition and membrane microviscosity in infants with atopic dermatitis. *Drugs Exp Clin Res* 20(2): 77–84, 1994.

Gallstones

1. Somerville KW, et al. Stones in the common bile duct: experience with medical dissolution therapy. *Postgrad Med J* 61: 313–316, 1985.

2. Nassauto G, et al. Effect of silibinin on biliary lipid composition: experimental and clinical study. *J Hepatol* 12: 290–295, 1991.

3. Schulz V, et al. Rational phytotherapy. New York: Springer-Verlag, 1998: 173–177.

Gout

1. Lewis AS, et al. Inhibition of mammalian xanthine oxidase by folate compounds and amethopterin. *J Biol Chem* 259: 12–15, 1984.
2. Blouvier B and Duvulder B. Folic acid, xanthine oxidase, and uric acid (Letter). *Ann Intern Med* 88(2): 269, 1978.
3. Boss GR, et al. Failure of folic acid (pteroylglutamic acid) to affect hyperuricemia. *J Lab Clin Med* 96: 783, 1980.
4. ESCOP monographs. Fascicule 2: *Harpagophyti radix*. Exeter, UK: European Scientific Cooperative on Phytotherapy, 1997: 4.
5. Murray, M. Encyclopedia of natural medicine, 2nd ed. Rocklin, CA: Prima Publishing, 1997: 493–94.
6. Blau LW. Cherry diet control for gout and arthritis. *Texas Rep Biol Med* 8: 309–312, 1950.

Hemorrhoids

1. Wijayanegara H, et al. A clinical trial of hydroxyethylrutosides in the treatment of hemorrhoids of pregnancy. *J Int Med Res* 20: 54–60, 1992.
2. Boisseau MR, et al. Fibrinolysis and hemorrheology in chronic venous insufficiency: a double-blind study of troxerutin efficiency. *J Cardiovasc Surg* 36: 369–374, 1995.
3. Wadworth AN, et al. Hydroxyethylrutosides: a review of its pharmacology and therapeutic efficacy in venous insufficiency and related disorders. *Drugs* 44: 1013–1032, 1992.
4. Saggloro A, et al. Treatment of hemorrhoidal syndrome with mesoglycan. *Minerva Diet Gastroenterol* 31: 311–315, 1985.
5. Annoni R, et al. Treatment of hemorrhoidal syndrome with mesoglycan. *Minerva Diet Gastroenterol* 31: 311–315, 1985.

Hepatitis

1. Berenguer J, et al. Double-blind trial of silymarin vs. placebo in the treatment of chronic hepatitis. *Muench Med Wochenschr* 119: 240–260, 1977.
2. Buzzelli G, et al. A pilot study on the liver protective effect of silybin-phosphatidylcholine complex (IdB1016) in chronic active hepatitis. *Int J Clin Pharm Ther Toxicol* 31(9): 456–460, 1993.
3. Liruss F, et al. Cytoprotection in the nineties: experience with ursodeoxycholic acid and silymarin in chronic liver disease. *Acta Physiol Hung* 80(1–4): 363–367, 1992.
4. Bode JC, et al. Silymarin for the treatment of acute viral hepatitis? Report of a controlled trial. *Med Klin* 72: 513–518, 1977.
5. Schulz V, et al. Rational phytotherapy. New York: Springer-Verlag, 1998: 216.
6. Hikino H, et al. Natural products for liver disease. As cited in Wagner H, et al. (eds.). Economic and medicinal plant research, Vol 2. New York: Academic Press, 1988: 39–72.
7. Muzes G, et al. Effects of silymarin (Legalon) therapy on the antioxidant defense mechanism and lipid peroxidation in alcoholic liver disease (double-blind protocol). *Orv Hetil* 131(16): 863–866, 1990.
8. Lorenz D, et al. Pharmacokinetic studies with silymarin in human serum and bile. *Methods Find Exp Clin Pharmacol* 6(10): 655–661, 1984.
9. Dehmlow C, et al. Inhibition of kupffer cell functions as an explanation for the hepatoprotective properties of silibinin. *Hepatology* 23(4): 749–754, 1996.
10. Comoglio A, et al. Scavenging effect of silipide, a new silybin-phospholipid complex, on ethanol-derived free radicals. *Biochem Pharmacol* 50(8): 1313–1316, 1995.
11. Barzaghi N, et al. Pharmacokinetic studies on IdB 1016, a silybin-phosphatidylcholine complex in healthy human subjects. *Eur J Drug Metab Pharmacokinet* 15(4): 333–338, 1990.
12. Schandalik R, et al. Pharmacokinetics of silybin in bile following administration of silipide and silymarin in cholecystectomy patients. *Arzneimittelforschung* 42(7): 964–968, 1992.
13. Awang D. Milk thistle. *Can Pharm J* 422: 403–404, 1983.

14. Albrecht M. Therapy of toxic liver pathologies with Legalon. *Z Klin Med* 47(2): 87–92, 1992.

15. Giannola C, et al. A two-center study on the effects of silymarin in pregnant women and adult patients with so-called minor hepatic insufficiency. *Clin Ther* 114(2): 129–135, 1985.

16. Kim DH, et al. Silymarin and its components are inhibitors of beta-glucuronidase. *Biol Pharm Bull* 17(3): 443–445, 1994.

17. Arase Y, et al. The long term efficacy of glycyrrhizin in chronic hepatitis C patients. *Cancer* 79: 1494–1500, 1997.

18. Okumura M, et al. A multicenter randomized controlled clinical trial of Sho-saiko-to in chronic active hepatitis. *Gastroenterol Jpn* 24: 715–719, 1989.

Herpes

1. Wolbling RH, et al. Local therapy of herpes simplex with dried extract from *Melissa officinalis*. *Phytomedicine* 1: 25–31, 1994.

2. Wolbling RH, et al. Clinical therapy of herpes simplex. *Therapiewoche* 34: 1193–1200, 1984.

3. Wolbling RH, et al., 1994.

4. Flodin NW. The metabolic roles, pharmacology, and toxicology of lysine. *J Am Coll Nutr* 16(1): 7–21, 1997.

5. Griffith RS, Walsh DE, and Myrmel KH. Success of L-lysine therapy in frequently recurrent herpes simplex infection. Treatment and prophylaxis. *Dermatologica*, 175: 183–190, 1987.

6. McCune MA, Perry HO, Muller SA, et al. Treatment of recurrent herpes simplex infections with L-lysine monohydrochloride. *Cutis* 34: 366–373, 1984.

7. DiGiovanna JJ and Blank H. Failure of lysine in frequently recurrent herpes simplex infection: treatment and prophylaxis. *Arch Dermatol* 120: 48–51, 1984.

8. Kritchevsky D, et al. Gallstone formation in hamsters: influence of specific amino acids. *Nutr Rep Int* 29: 117, 1984.

9. Lexzczynski DE, et al. Excess dietary lysine induces hypercholesterolemia in chickens. *Experientia* 38: 266–267, 1982.

10. Hovi T, et al. Topical treatment of recurrent mucocutaneous herpes with ascorbic acid–containing solution. *Antiviral Res* 27(3): 263–270, 1995.

11. Terezhalmy GT, Bottomley WK, and Pelleu GB. The use of water-soluble bioflavonoid-ascorbic acid complex in the treatment of recurrent herpes labialis. *Oral Surg Oral Med Oral Pathol* 45(1): 56–62, 1978.

Hypertension

1. Silagy CA, et al. A meta-analysis of the effect of garlic on blood pressure. *J Hypertens* 12: 463–468, 1994.

2. Auer W, et al. Hypertension and hyperlipidemia: garlic helps in mild cases. *Br J Clin Pract Symp Suppl* 69: 3–6, 1990.

3. Digiesi V, et al. Effect of coenzyme Q_{10} on essential arterial hypertension. *Curr Ther Res* 47: 841–845, 1990.

4. Appel LJ, et al. Does supplementation of diet with "fish oil" reduce blood pressure? A meta-analysis of controlled clinical trials. *Arch Intern Med* 153(12): 1429–1438, 1993.

5. McCarron DA, et al. Dietary calcium and blood pressure: modifying factors in specific populations. *Am J Clin Nutr* 54: 215S–219S, 1991.

6. Bucher HC, Cook RJ, Guyatt GH, et al. Effects of dietary calcium supplementation on blood pressure. *JAMA* 275(13): 1016–1022, 1996.

7. Altura BM and Altura BT. Cardiovascular risk factors and magnesium: relationships to atherosclerosis, ischemic heart disease and hypertension. *Magnes Trace Elements* 10: 182–192, 1991.

8. Ma J, Folsom AR, Melnick SL, et al. Associations of serum and dietary magnesium with cardiovascular disease, hypertension, diabetes, insulin and carotid artery wall thickness: the ARIC study. *J Clin Epidemiol* 48(7): 927–940, 1995.

9. Yamamoto ME, Applegate WB, Klag MJ, et al. Lack of blood pressure effect with calcium and magnesium supplementation in adults with high-normal blood pressure: Results from phase I of the trials of hypertension prevention (TOHP). *Ann Epidemiol* 5: 96–107, 1995.

10. Barri YM and Wingo CS. The effects of potassium depletion and supplementation on blood pressure: a clinical review. *Am J Med Sci* 314(1): 37–40, 1997.

11. Whelton PK, He J, Cutler JA, et al. Effects of oral potassium on blood pressure. Meta-analysis of randomized controlled clinical trials. *JAMA* 277(20): 1624–1632, 1997.

12. Preuss HG. Diet, genetics and hypertension. *J Am Coll Nutr* 16(4): 296–305, 1997.

13. Schulz V, et al. Rational phytotherapy. New York: Springer-Verlag, 1998: 97.

14. Osilesi O, et al. Blood pressure and plasma lipids during ascorbic acid supplementation in borderline hypertensive and normotensive adults. *Nutr Res* 11: 405–412, 1991.

15. Feldman E, Gold S, Green J, et al. Ascorbic acid supplements and blood pressure. *Ann NY Acad Sci* 669: 342–344, 1992.

16. Feldman EB, Gold S, Greene J, et al. Vitamin C administration and blood pressure regulation (Abstract). *Am J Clin Nutr* 56: 760, 1992.

17. Koh ET. Effect of vitamin C on blood parameters of hypertensive subjects. *J Okla State Med Assoc* 77: 177–182, 1984.

18. Ghosh S, Ekpo E, and Shah I. A double-blind, placebo-controlled parallel trial of vitamin C treatment in elderly patients with hypertension. *Gerontology* 40: 268–272, 1994.

Impotence

1. Sikora R, et al. *Ginkgo biloba* extract in the therapy of erectile dysfunction. *J Urol* 141: 188A, 1989.

2. Cohen AJ and Bartlik B. *Ginkgo biloba* for antidepressant-induced sexual dysfunction. *J Sex Marital Ther* 24: 139–143, 1988.

Infertility in Men

1. Werbach, M. Nutritional influences on illness, 2nd ed. Tarzana, CA: Third Line Press, 1993: 628–629.

2. Kumamoto Y, et al. Clinical efficacy of mecobalamin in treatment of oligozoospermia: Results of double-blind comparative clinical study. *Acta Urol Jpn* 34: 1109–1132, 1988.

3. Sandler B, and Faragher B. Treatment of oligospermia with vitamin B$_{12}$. *Infertility* 7: 133–138, 1984.

4. Bedwal R, et al. Zinc, copper and selenium in reproduction. *Experientia* 50: 626–640, 1994.

5. Netter A, et al. Effect of zinc administration on plasma testosterone, dihydrotestosterone and sperm count. *Arch Androl* 7: 69–73, 1981.

6. Suleiman SA, Ali ME, Zaki ZM, et al. Lipid peroxidation and human sperm motility: protective role of vitamin E. *J Androl* 17(5): 530–537, 1996.

7. Dawson EB, et al. Effect of ascorbic acid on male fertility. *Ann NY Acad Sci* 498: 312–323, 1987.

Infertility in Women

1. Propping D, et al. Diagnosis and therapy of corpus luteum insufficiency in general practice. *Therapiewoche* 38: 2992–3001, 1988.

2. Czeizel A, Metnek J, and Dudas I. The effect of preconceptional multivitamin supplementation on fertility. *Int J Vitam Nutr Res* 66: 55–58, 1996.

Insomnia

1. Schulz V, et al. Rational phytotherapy. New York: Springer-Verlag, 1998: 75–77, 81.

2. Hendriks H, et al. Central nervous depressant activity of valerenic acid in the mouse. *Planta Medica* 51: 28–31, 1985.

3. Krieglstein J, et al. Valepotriate, valenrensaure, valeranon und atherisches Ol sind jedoch unwirksam. Zentraldampfende Inhaltsstoffe im Baldrian. *Dtsch Apoth Ztg* 128: 2041–2046, 1988.

4. Leuschner J, et al. Characterization of the central nervous depressant activity of a commercially available valerian root extract. *Arzneimittelforschung* 43(6): 638–641, 1993.

5. Vorbach EU, et al. Therapie von Insomnien. Wirksamkeit und Vertraglichkeit eines Baldrianpraparats. *Psychopharmakotherapie* 3: 109–115, 1996. As cited in Schulz V, et al., Rational phytotherapy. New York: Springer-Verlag, 1998.

6. Leathwood PD, et al. Aqueous extract of valerian root *(Valeriana officinalis* L.) improves sleep quality in man. *Pharmacol Biochem Behav* 17(1): 65–71, 1982.

7. Leathwood PD, et al. Aqueous extract of valerian reduces latency to fall asleep in man. *Planta Medica* 51: 144–148, 1985.

8. Lindahl O, et al. Double-blind study of a valerian preparation. *Pharmacol Biochem Behav* 32(4): 1065–1066, 1989.

9. Kamm-Khol AV, et al. Moderne Baldriantherapie gegen nervose Storungen im Senium. *Med Welt* 35: 1450–1454, 1985. As cited in ESCOP monographs. Fascicule 4: *Valerianae radix* (valerian root) Exeter, UK: European Society Cooperative on Phytotherapy, 1997.

10. Andreatini R and Leite JR. Effect of valepotriates on the behavior of rats in the elevated plus-maze during diazepam withdrawal. *Eur J Pharmacol* 260(2–3): 233–235, 1994.

11. Holzl J, et al. Receptor binding studies with *Valeriana officinalis* on the benzodiazepine receptor. *Planta Medica* 55: 642, 1989.

12. Mennini T, et al. In vitro study on the interaction of extracts and pure compounds from *Valeriana officinalis* roots with GABA, benzodiazepine and barbiturate receptors in rat brain. *Fitoterapia* 54: 291–300, 1993.

13. Santos MS, et al. Synaptosomal GABA release as influenced by valerian root extract—involvement of the GABA carrier. *Arch Int Pharmacodyn* 327: 220–231, 1994.

14. Santos MS, et al. An aqueous extract of valerian influences the transport of GABA in synaptosomes. *Planta Medica* 60: 278–279, 1994.

15. Cavadas C, et al. In vitro study on the interaction of *Valeriana officinalis* L: Extracts and their amino acids on GABA receptor in rat brain. *Arznemittelforschung* 45(7): 753–755, 1995.

16. Santos MS, et al. The amount of GABA present in aqueous extracts of valerian is sufficient to account for [^{3}H] GABA release in synaptosomes. *Planta Medica* 60: 475–476, 1994.

17. Schulz V, et al., 1998.

18. Wiley LB, et al. Valerian overdose: a case report. *Vet Hum Toxicol* 37(4): 364–365, 1995.

19. Rosecrans JA, et al. Pharmacological investigation of certain *Valeriana officinalis* L. extracts. *J Pharm Sci* 50: 240–244, 1996.

20. Schulz V, et al., 1998.

21. Albrecht M, et al. Psychopharmaceuticals and safety in traffic. *Z Allg Med* 71: 1215–1221, 1995.

22. Gerhard U, et al. Vigilance-decreasing effects of 2 plant-derived sedatives. *Schweiz Rundsch Med Prax* 85(15): 473–481, 1996.

23. Sakamoto T, et al. Psychotropic effects of Japanese valerian root extract. *Chem Pharm Bull (Tokyo)* 40(3): 758–761, 1992.

24. Albrecht M. et al., 1995.

25. Lamberg L. Melatonin potentially useful but safety, efficacy remain uncertain. *JAMA* 276(13): 1011–1014, 1996.

26. Suhner A, et al. Optimal melatonin dosage form for the alleviation of jet lag. *Chronobiol Int* 14: 41, 1997.

27. Garfinkel D, et al. Improvement of sleep quality in elderly people by controlled-release melatonin. *Lancet* 346: 541–544, 1995.

28. Petrie K, et al. A double-blind trial of melatonin as a treatment for jet lag in international cabin crew. *Biol Psych* 33(7): 526–530, 1993.

29. Chase JE, et al. Melatonin: therapeutic use in sleep disorders. *Ann Pharmacother* 346(10): 1218–1226, 1997.

30. Spitzer RL, et al. Failure of melatonin to affect jet lag in a randomized double-blind trial. *Soc Light Treatment Biol Rhythms Abstr* 9: 1, 1997.

31. Arendt J, et al. Efficacy of melatonin in jet lag, shift work and blindness. *J Biol Rhythms* 12(6): 604–617, 1997.

32. Suhner A, et al., 1997.

33. Waterhouse J, et al. Jet lag. *Lancet* 350: 1611–1616, 1997.

Intermittent Claudication

1.Schulz V, et al. Rational phytotherapy. New York: Springer-Verlag, 1998: 126.

2. Peters H, Kieser M, and Holscher U. Demonstration of the efficacy of *Ginkgo biloba* special extract EGb 761 on intermittent claudication—a placebo-controlled, double-blind multicenter trial. *Vasa* 27: 106–110, 1998.

3. Blume J, Kieser M, and Holscher U. Placebo-controlled double-blind study of the effectiveness of *Ginkgo biloba* special extract EGb 761 in trained patients with intermittent claudication (Engl Abst Only). *Vasa* 25: 265–274, 1996.

4. Peters H, Kieser M, and Holscher U., 1998.

5. Brevetti G, et al. Propionyl-L-carnitine in intermittent claudication: double-blind, placebo-controlled, dose titration, multicenter study. *J Am Coll Cardiol* 26(6): 1411–1416, 1995.

Irritable Bowel Syndrome

1. Rees WDW, et al. Treating irritable bowel syndrome with peppermint oil. *BMJ* 2: 835–836, 1979.

2. Dew MJ, et al. Peppermint oil for the irritable bowel syndrome: A multicentre trial. *Br J Clin Pract* 34: 55–57, 1989.

3. Lawson MJ, et al. Failure of enteric-coated peppermint oil in the irritable bowel syndrome: A randomized double-blind crossover study. *J Gastroenterol Hepatol* 3: 235–238, 1988.

4. Nash P, et al. Peppermint oil does not relieve the pain of irritable bowel syndrome. *Br J Clin Pract* 40: 292–293, 1986.

5. ESCOP monographs. Fascicule 3: *Menthae piperitae aetheroleum* (peppermint oil). Exeter, UK: European Scientific Cooperative on Phytotherapy, 1997: 1–2.

Macular Degeneration

1. Mares-Perlman J, Klein R, Klein B, et al. Relationship between age-related maculopathy and intake of vitamin and mineral supplements (Abstract). *Invest Ophthalmol Vis Sci* 34: 1133, 1993.

2. Mares-Perlman JA, et al. Association of zinc and antioxidant nutrients with age-related maculopathy. *Arch Ophthalmol* 114: 991–997, 1996.

3. Age-Related Macular Degeneration Study Group. Multicenter ophthalmic and nutritional age-related macular degeneration study—Part 2: antioxidant intervention and conclusions. *J Am Optom Assoc* 67: 30–49, 1996.

4. Seddon JM, Ajani UA, Sperduto RD, et al. Dietary carotenoids, vitamins A, C, and E, and advanced age-related macular degeneration. *JAMA* 272: 1413–1420, 1994.

5. Mares-Perlman JA, Brady W, Klein R, et al. Serum antioxidants and age-related macular degeneration in a population-based case-control study. *Arch Ophthalmol* 113: 1518–1523, 1995.

6. Landrum JT, Bone RA, and Kilburn MD. The macular pigment: a possible role in protection from age-related macular degeneration. *Adv Pharmacol* 38: 537–555, 1997.

7. Snodderly DM. Evidence for protection against age-related macular degeneration by carotenoids and antioxidant vitamins. *Am J Clin Nutr* 62(14): 48S–61S, 1995.

8. Scharrer A, et al. Anthocyanosides in the treatment of retinopathies. *Klin Monatsbl Augenheilkd* 178: 386–389, 1981.

9. Lebuisson DA, et al. Treatment of senile macular degeneration with *Ginkgo biloba* extract: A preliminary double-blind, drug vs. placebo study. *Presse Med* 15: 1556–1558, 1986.

10. Caselli L. Clinical and electroretinographic study on activity of anthocyanosides. *Arch Med Int* 37: 29–35, 1985.

11. Watson V. Wine consumption decreases risk of age-related blindness. *Medical Tribune*, June 5, 1997.

12. Stur M, et al. Oral zinc and the second eye in age-related macular degeneration. *Invest Ophthalmol Visual Sci* 37(7): 1225–1235, 1996.

13. Mares-Perlman JA, et al., 1996.

14. Newsome DA, Swartz M, Leone NC, et al. Oral zinc in macular degeneration. *Arch Ophthalmol* 106(2): 192–198, 1988.

Menopausal Symptoms

1. Stoll W. Phythopharmacon influences atrophic vaginal epithelium. Double-blind study: Cimicifuga vs. estrogenic substances. *Therapeuticum* 1: 23–28, 1987.

2. Stolze H. An alternative to treat menopausal complaints. *Gyne* 3: 14–16, 1982.

3. Warnecke G. Influencing menopausal symptoms with a phytotherapeutic agent. *Med Welt* 36: 871–874, 1985.

4. Stoll W., 1987.

5. Stolze H., 1982.

6. Warnecke G., 1985.

7. Jarry H, et al. The endocrine effects of constituents of *Cimicifuga racemosa*. 2. In vitro binding of constituents to estrogen receptors. *Planta Medica* 4: 316–319, 1985.

8. Jarry H, et al. Endocrine effects of constituents of *Cimicifuga racemosa*. 1. The effect on serum levels of pituitary hormones in ovariectomized rats. *Planta Medica* 1: 46–49, 1985.

9. Duker EM, et al. Effects of extracts from *Cimicifuga racemosa* on gonadotropin release in menopausal women and ovariectomized rats. *Planta Medica* 57(5): 420–424, 1991.

10. Schaper & Brümmer. Remifemin®: a plant-based gynecological agent. Scientific brochure, 1997.

11. Jones TK, et al. Profound neonatal congestive heart failure caused by maternal consumption of blue cohosh herbal medication. *J Pediatrics* 132: 550–552, 1998.

12. Korn WD. Six-month oral toxicity study with Remifemin-granulate in rats followed by an 8-week recovery period. Hannover, Germany: International Bio-research, 1991.

13. Nesselhut T, et al. Influence of *Cimicifuga racemosa* extracts with estrogen-like activity on the in vitro proliferation of mammalian carcinoma cells. *Arch Gynecol Obstet* 254: 817–818, 1993.

14. Newall C. Herbal medicines: a guide for the health-care professional. London: The Pharmaceutical Press, 1996: 80.

15. Albertazzi P, et al. The effect of dietary soy supplementation on hot flashes. *Obstet Gynecol* 91(1): 6–11, 1998.

16. Hughes C. Complementary medicine for the physician. 3(4): 26–27, 1998.

17. Messina M. To recommend or not to recommend soy foods. *J Am Diet Assoc* 94(11): 1253–1254.

18. Hirata JD, et al. Does dong quai have estrogenic effects in postmenopausal women? A double-blind placebo-controlled trial. *Fertil Steril* 68(6): 981–986, 1997.

Migraine Headaches

1. Johnson ES, et al. Efficacy of feverfew as a prophylactic treatment of migraine. *BMJ* 291: 569–573, 1983.

2. Murphy JS, et al. Randomized, double-blind, placebo-controlled trial of feverfew in migraine prevention. *Lancet* 23: 189–192, 1988.

3. Palevitch DG, et al. Feverfew *(Tanacetum parthenium)* as a prophylactic treatment for migraine: A double-blind, placebo controlled study. *Phytother Res* 11(7): 506–511, 1997.

4. De Weerdt C, et al. Herbal medicines in migraine prevention. Randomized double-blind placebo controlled crossover trial of a feverfew preparation. *Phytomedicine* 3(3): 225–230, 1996.

5. Bohlmann F, et al. Sesquiterpene lactones and other constituents from *Tanacetum parthenium. Phytochemistry* 21: 2543–2549, 1982.

6. Makheja AM, et al. The active principle in feverfew. *Lancet* ii: 1054, 1981.

7. Makheja AM, et al. A platelet phospholipase inhibitor from the medicinal herb feverfew *(Tanacetum parthenium). Prostaglandins Leukotriens Med* 8: 653–660, 1982.

8. Heptinstall S, et al. Extracts from feverfew inhibit granule secretion in blood platelets and polymorphonuclear leukocytes. *Lancet* 8437: 1071–1074, 1985.

9. Tyler V. Herbs of choice. New York: Pharmaceutical Products Press, 1994: 127.

10. Murphy JS, et al., 1988.

11. Johnson ES, et al., 1985.

12. Johnson ES, et al., 1985.

13. Newall C, et al. Herbal medicines: a guide for health-care professionals. London: The Pharmaceutical Press, 1996: 120.

14. Peikert A, et al. Prophylaxis of migraine with oral magnesium: results from a prospective, multi-center, placebo-controlled and double-blind randomized study. *Cephalalgia* 6(4): 257–263, 1996.

15. Taubert K. Magnesium in migraine: Results of a multicenter pilot study (in German). *Fortschr Med* 112(24): 328–330, 1994.

16. Facchinetti F, Sances G, Borella P, et al. Magnesium prophylaxis of menstrual migraine: effects on intracellular magnesium. *Headache* 31(5): 298–301, 1991.

17. Pfaffenrath V, et al. Magnesium in the prophylaxis of migraine—a double-blind, placebo-controlled study. *Cephalalgia* 16: 436–440, 1996.

18. Gaby AR. Research Review. *Nutrition & Healing,* March 1997.

19. Titus F, et al. 5-hydroxytryptophan versus methysergide in the prophylaxis of migraine: randomized clinical trial. *Eur Neurol* 25(5): 327–329, 1986.

20. De Benedittis G and Massei R. Serotonin precursors in chronic primary headache. A double-blind cross-over study with L-5-hydroxytryptophan vs. placebo. *J Neurosurg Sci* 29(3): 239–248, 1985.

21. Maissen CP and Ludin HP. Comparison of the effect of 5-hydroxytryptophan and propranolol in the interval treatment of migraine. *Schweiz Med Wochenschr* 121(43): 1585–1590, 1991.

22. Longo G, Rudoi I, Iannuccelli M, et al. Treatment of essential headache in developmental age with L-5-HTP (crossover double-blind study versus placebo). *Pediatr Med Chir* 6(2): 241–245, 1984.

23. Santucci M, et al. L-hydroxytryptophan versus placebo in childhood migraine prophylaxis: a double-blind crossover study. *Cephalalgia* 6: 155–157, 1986.

24. Glueck CJ, et al. Amelioration of severe migraine with omega-3 fatty acids: A double-blind, placebo-controlled clinical trial (Abstract). *Am J Clin Nutr* 43: 710, 1986.

25. Macaroon T, et al. Amelioration of severe migraine by fish oil (w-3) fatty acids (Abstract). *Am J Clin Nutr* 41: 874a, 1985.

26. Trotsky MB. Neurogenic vascular headaches, food and chemical triggers. *Ear Nose Throat J* 73(4): 228–230, 235–236, 1994.

27. Vincent CA. A controlled trial of the treatment of migraine by acupuncture. *Clin J Pain* 5(4): 305–312, 1989.

Nausea

1. Fischer-Rasmussen W, et al. Ginger treatment of hyperemesis gravidarum. *Eur J Obstet Gynecol Reprod Biol* 38: 19–24, 1990.

2. Mowrey DB. Motion sickness, ginger, and psychophysics. *Lancet* i: 655–657, 1982.

3. ESCOP monographs. Fascicule 1: *Zingiberis rhizoma* (ginger). Exeter, UK: European Scientific Cooperative on Phytotherapy, 1997: 2.

4. Grontved A, et al. Ginger root against seasickness: A controlled trial on the open sea. *Acta Otolaryngol (Stockh)* 105: 45–49, 1988.

5. Stott JRR, et al. A double-blind comparative trial of powdered ginger root, hyosine (sic) hydrobromide and cinnarizine in the prophylaxis of motion sickness induced by cross coupled stimulation. *Advisory Group for Aerospace Research and Development, Conference Proceedings* 372(39): 1–6, 1985.

6. Stewart JJ, et al. Effects of ginger on motion sickness susceptibility and gastric function. *Pharmacology* 42: 111–120, 1991.

7. Bone ME, Wilkinson DJ, Young JR, et al. Ginger root: a new anti-emetic. The effect of ginger root on postoperative nausea and vomiting after major gynecological surgery. *Anaesthesia* 45: 669–671, 1990.

8. Phillips S, et al. *Zingiber officinale* (ginger)—an anti-emetic for day case surgery. *Anaesthesia* 48: 715–717, 1993.

9. Arfeen Z, et al. A double-blind randomized controlled trial of ginger for the prevention of postoperative nausea and vomiting. *Anaesth Intensive Care* 23 (4): 449–452, 1995.

10. Visalyaputra S, et al. The efficacy of ginger root in the prevention of postoperative nausea and vomiting after outpatient gynaecological laparoscopy. *Anaesthesia* 53: 506–510, 1998.

11. Janssen PL, et al. Consumption of ginger (*Zingiber officinale* Roscoe) does not affect ex vivo platelet thromboxane production in humans. *Eur J Clin Nutr* 50(11): 772–774, 1996.

12. Bordia A, et al. Effect of ginger (*Zingiber officinale* Rosc.) and fenugreek (*Trigonella foenumgraecum* L.) on blood lipids, blood sugar and platelet aggregation in patients with coronary artery disease. *Prostaglandins Leukot Essent Fatty Acids* 56(5): 379–384, 1997.

13. Lumb AB. Effect of dried ginger on human platelet function. *Thromb Haemost* 71: 110–111, 1994.

14. Merkel RL. The use of menadione bisulfite and ascorbic acid in the treatment of nausea and vomiting of pregnancy. *Am J Obstet Gynecol* 78: 33–36, 1952.

15. Signorello LB, et al. Saturated fat intake and the risk of severe hyperemesis gravidarum. *Am J Epidemiol* 143(Suppl. 11): S25, 1996.

Night Vision

1. Jayle GE, et al. Action des glucosides d'anthocyanes sur la vision scotopique et mesopique du sujet normal. *Therapie* 19: 171–185, 1964. As cited in Bone K, et al., *Mediherb Professional Review*. Queensland, Australia, 59, 1997.

2. Jayle GE, et al.. Title not stated. *Ann Ocul* 198: 556, 1965. As cited in Bone K, et al., *Mediherb Professional Review*. Queensland, Australia, 59, 1997.

3. Sala D, et al. Effect of anthocyanosides on visual performance at low illumination. *Minerva Oftalmol* 21: 283–285, 1979.

4. Gloria E, et al. Effect of anthocyanosides on the absolute visual threshold. *Ann Ottalmol Clin Ocul* 92: 595–607, 1966.

5. Caselli L. Clinical and electroretinographic study on activity of anthocyanosides. *Arch Med Int* 37: 29–35, 1985.

6. Wegmann R, et al. Effects of anthocyanosides on photoreceptors. Cyto-enzymatic aspects. *Ann Histochem* 14: 237–256, 1969.

7. Lietti A, et al. Studies on *Vaccinium myrtillus* anthocyanosides: vasoprotective and anti-inflammatory activity. *Arzneimittelforschung* 26: 829–832, 1976.

8. Lietti A, et al. Studies on *Vaccinium myrtillus* anthocyanosides: aspects of antho-cyanin pharmacokinetics in the rat. *Arzneimittelforschung* 26: 832–835, 1976.

9. Eandi M. Unpublished results. As cited in Morazzoni P, et al., *Vaccinium myrtillus*. *Fitoterapia* 67(1): 3–29 1996.

Osteoarthritis

1. Brandt KD. Effects of nonsteroidal anti-inflammatory drugs on chondrocyte metabolism in vitro and in vivo. *Am J Med* 83 (Suppl. 5A): 29–34, 1987.

2. Brooks PM, et al. NSAID and osteoarthritis—help or hindrance. *J Rheumatol* 9: 3–5, 1982.

3. Shield MJ, Anti-inflammatory drugs and their effects on cartilage synthesis and renal function. *Eur J Rheumatol Inflam* 13: 7–16, 1993.

4. Palmoski MJ, et al. Effects of some nonsteroidal anti-inflammatory drugs on proteoglycan metabolism and organization in canine articular cartilage. *Arthritis Rheum* 23: 1010–1020, 1980.

5. Rahad S, et al. Effects of nonsteroidal anti-inflammatory drugs on the course of osteoarthritis. *Lancet* 2: 519–522, 1989.

6. Jimenez SA, et al. The effects of glucosamine on human chondrocyte gene expres-sion. Madrid, Spain: The Ninth Eular Symposium, 1996: 8–10.

7. Hellio MP, et al. The effects of glucosamine on human chondrocyte gene expres-sion. Madrid, Spain: The Ninth Eular Symposium, 1996: 11–12.

8. Setnikar I, et al. Anti-arthritic effects of glucosamine sulfate studied in animal models. *Arzneim Forsch* 41: 542–545, 1991.

9. Setnikar I. Antireactive properties of "chondroprotective" drugs. *Int J Tissue React* 14(5): 253–261, 1992.

10. Crolle G, et al. Glucosamine sulfate for the management of arthrosis: A controlled clinical investigation. *Current Medical Research and Opinion* 7(2): 104–109, 1980.

11. Qiu GX, et al. Efficacy and safety of glucosamine sulfate versus ibuprofen in patients with knee arthritis. *Arzneimittelforschung* 48: 469–474, 1998.

12. Karzel K, et al. Effect of hexosamine derivatives and uronic acid derivatives on glycosaminoglycan metabolism of fibroblast cultures. *Pharmacology* 5: 337–345, 1971.

13. Vidal y Plana, et al. Articular cartilage pharmacology: I. In vitro studies on glu-cosamine and nonsteroidal anti-inflammatory drugs. *Pharmacol Res Comm* 10: 557–569, 1978.

14. Noack W, et al. Glucosamine sulfate in osteoarthritis of the knee. *Osteoarthritis Cartilage* 2: 51–59, 1994.

15. Rovati, LC, et al. A large, randomized, placebo controlled, double-blind study of glucosamine sulfate vs. Piroxicam and vs. their association, on the kinetics of the symptomatic effect in knee osteoarthritis. *Osteoarthritis Cartilage* 2(Suppl. 1): 56, 1994.

16. Muller-Fassbender H, et al. Glucosamine sulfate compared to ibuprofen in osteoarthritis of the knee. *Osteoarthritis Cartilage* 2: 61–69, 1994.

17. Qiu GX, et al., 1998.

18. Setnikar I, et al. Pharmacokinetics of glucosamine in man. *Arzneimittelforschung* 43(10): 1109–1113, 1993.

19. Tapadinhas MJ, et al. Oral glucosamine sulfate in the management of arthrosis: Report on multi-centre open investigation in Portugal. *Pharmatherapeutica* 3: 157–168, 1982.

20. Conte A, et al. Biochemical and pharmacokinetic aspects of oral treatment with chondroitin sulfate. *Arzneim Forsch Drug Res* 45: 918–925, 1995.

21. Hungerford, DS. Treating osteoarthritis with chondroprotective agents. *Ortho-pedic Special Edition* 4(1): 39–42, 1998.

22. Busci L and Poor G. Efficacy and tolerability of oral chondroitin sulfate as a symptomatic slow-acting drug for osteoarthritis (SYSADOA) in the treatment of knee osteoarthritis. *Osteoarthritis and Cartilage* 6(Suppl. A): 31–36, 1998.

23. Bourgeois R, Chales G, Dehais J, et al. Efficacy and tolerability of CS 1,200 mg/day versus CS 3x400 mg/day versus placebo. *Osteoarthritis and Cartilage* 6(Suppl. A): 25–30, 1998.

24. Uebelhart D, et al. Protective effect of exogenous chondroitin 4,6-sulfate in the acute degradation of articular cartilage in the rabbit. *Osteoarthritis and Cartilage* 6(Suppl. A): 6–13, 1998.

25. Verbruggen G, Goemaere S, and Veys EM. Chondroitin sulfate: S/DMOAD (structure/disease modifying anti osteoarthritis drug) in the treatment of finger joint OA. *Osteoarthritis and Cartilage* 6(Suppl. A): 37–38, 1998.

26. Uebelhart D, et al., 1998.

27. di Padova C. S-adenosylmethionine in the treatment of osteoarthritis: Review of the clinical studies. *Am J Med* 83(Suppl. 5A): 60–65, 1989.

28. Caruso I and Peitrogrande V. Italian double-blind multicenter study comparing S-adenosylmethionine, naproxen, and placebo in the treatment of degenerative joint disease. *Am J Med* 83(Suppl. 5A): 66–71, 1987.

29. Kalbhen DA, et al. Pharmakologische Untersuchungen zur antidegenerativen Wirkung von Ademetionin bei der tierexperimentellen Arthrose. *Arzneimittelforschung* 40(9): 1017–1021.

30. Barcelo HA, et al. Experimental osteoarthritis and its course when treated with S-adenyl-L-methionine. *Rev Clin Esp* 187(2): 74–78, 1990.

31. Cozens DD, et al. Reproductive toxicity studies of ademetionine. *Arzneimittelforschung* 38(11): 1625–1629, 1988.

32. Berger R, et al. A new medical approach to the treatment of osteoarthritis: Report of an open phase IV study with ademethionine (Gumbaral). *Am J Med* 83(Suppl 5A): 84–88, 1987.

33. Konig B. A long-term (two years) clinical trial with S-adenosylmethionine for the treatment of osteoarthritis. *Am J Med* 83(Suppl. 5A): 89–94, 1987.

34. Caruso I and Pietrogrande V., 1987.

35. di Padova C., 1989.

36. Carney MWP, et al. Switch and S-adenosylmethionine. *Ala J Med Sci* 25(3): 316–319, 1988.

37. Carney MWP, et al. The switch mechanism and the bipolar/unipolar dichotomy. *Br J Psych* 154: 48–51, 1989.

38. Cerutti R, et al. Psychological distress during peurperium: A novel therapeutic approach using S-adenosylmethionine. *Curr Ther Res* 53: 707–717, 1993.

39. Reicks M, et al. Effects of methionine and other sulfur compounds on drug conjugations. *Pharmacol Ther* 37: 67–79, 1988.

40. Iruela LM, et al. Toxic interaction of S-adenosylmethionine and clomipramine. *Am J Psych* 150: 522, 1993.

41. ESCOP monographs. Fascicule 2: *Harpagophyti radix* (devil's claw). Exeter, UK: European Scientific Cooperative on Phytotherapy, 1997: 4.

42. ESCOP monographs, 1997: 1–2.

43. ESCOP monographs, 1997.

44. McAlindon TE, et al. Do antioxidant micronutrients protect against the development and progression of knee OA? *Arth Rheum* 39: 648–656, 1996.

Osteoporosis

1. Reid IR. The roles of calcium and vitamin D in the prevention of osteoporosis. *Endocrinol Metab Clin North Am* 27: 389–398, 1998.

2. Cumming RG. Calcium intake and bone mass: A qualitative review of the evidence. *Calcif Tissue Int* 47: 194–201, 1990.

3. Dawson-Hughes B, Dallal GE, Krall EA, et al. A controlled trial of the effect of calcium supplementation on bone density in postmenopausal women. *N Engl J Med* 323(13): 878–883, 1990.

4. Prince R. Diet and the prevention of osteoporotic fractures. *N Engl J Med* 337(10): 701–702, 1997.

5. Nieves JW, et al. Calcium potentiates the effect of estrogen and calcitonin on bone mass: review and analysis. *Am J Clin Nutr* 67(1): 18–24, 1998.

6. Aloia JF, et al. Calcium supplementation with and without hormone replacement therapy to prevent postmenopausal bone loss. *Annals Intern Med* 120: 97–103, 1994.

7. Lloyd T, Andon MB, and Rollings N. Calcium supplementation and bone mineral density in adolescent girls. *JAMA* 270(7): 841–844, 1993.

8. Saltman PD, et al. The role of trace minerals in osteoporosis. *J Am Coll Nutr* 12(4): 384–389, 1993.

9. Strause L, et al. Spinal bone loss in postmenopausal women supplemented with calcium and trace minerals. *J Nutr* 124: 1060–1064, 1994.

10. Kruger MC, et al. Calcium, gamma-linolenic acid (GLA) and eicosapentaenoic acid (EPA) supplementation in osteoporosis. *Osteoporosis Int* 6(Suppl. 1): 250, 1996.

11. van Papendorp DH, Coetzer H, and Kruger MC. Biochemical profile of osteoporotic patients on essential fatty acid supplementation. *Nutr Res* 15(3): 325–334, 1995.

12. NIH Consensus Development Panel on Optimal Calcium Intake. *Nutrition* 11: 409–417, 1994.

13. Curhan GC, Willett WC, and Rimm EB. A prospective study of dietary calcium and supplemental calcium and other nutrients as factors affecting the risk of kidney stones in women. *Ann Int Med* 126: 497–504, 1997.

14. Curhan GC, Willett WC, and Rimm EB. A prospective study of dietary calcium and other nutrients and the risk of symptomatic kidney stones. *N Engl J Med* 328: 833–838, 1993.

15. Agnusdei D, et al. A double-blind placebo-controlled trial of ipiflavone for prevention of postmenopausal spinal bone loss. *Calcif Tissue Int* 61: 142–147, 1997.

16. Genari C, Adami S, Agusei L, et al. Effect of chronic treatment with ipriflavone in postmenopausal women with low bone mass. *Calcif Tissue Int* 61: S19–S22, 1997.

17. Valente, M. Bufalino L, et al. Effects of 1-year treatment with ipriflavone on bone in postmenopausal women with low bone mass. *Calcif Tissue Int* 54: 377–380, 1994.

18. Kovacs AB. Efficacy of ipriflavone in the prevention and treatment of postmenopausal osteoporosis. *Agents Actions* 41: 86–87, 1994.

19. Adami S, et al. Ipriflavone prevents radial bone loss in postmenopausal women with low bone mass over 2 years. *Osteoporos Int* 7(2): 119–125, 1997.

20. Agnusdei D, et al. Efficacy of ipriflavone in established osteoporosis and long-term safety. *Calcif Tissue Int* 61(1): S23–S27, 1997.

21. Agnusdei D, et al. A double-blind placebo-controlled trial of ipriflavone. 1997.

22. Agnusdei D, et al. Effects of ipriflavone on bone mass and bone remodeling in patients with established postmenopausal osteoporosis. *Curr Ther Res* 51(1): 82–91, 1992.

23. Gambacciani M, Cappagli B, Piaggesi M, et al. Ipriflavone prevents the loss of bone mass in pharmacological menopause produced by GnRH-agonists. *Calcif Tissue Int* 61: S15–S18, 1997.

24. Melis GB and Paoletti AM. Ipriflavone and low doses of estrogens in the prevention of bone mineral loss in climacterium. *Bone Mineral* 19: S49–S56, 1992.

25. Nozaki M, Hashimoto K, et al. Treatment of bone loss in ooporectomized women with a combination of ipriflavone and conjugated equine estrogen. *Int J Gyn Ob* 62: 69–75, 1998.

26. Agnusdei D and Bufalino L. Efficacy of ipriflavone in established osteoporosis and long-term safety. *Calcif Tissue Int* 61: S23–S27, 1997.

27. Melis G, Paoletti A, and Cagnacci A. Lack of any estrogenic effect of ipriflavone in postmenopausal women. *J Endrocrinol Invest* 15: 755–761, 1992.

28. Nielsen FH, et al. Effect of dietary boron on mineral, estrogen and testosterone metabolism in postmenopausal women. *FASEB J* 1: 394–397, 1987.

29. Naghii MR and Samman S. The effect of boron supplementation on its urinary excretion and selected cardiovascular risk factors in healthy male subjects. *Biol Trace Elem Res* 56(3): 273–286, 1997.

30. Prior JC. Progesterone as a bone-trophic hormone. *Endocr Rev* 1: 386–398, 1986.

Periodontal Disease

1. Hanoika T, et al. Effect of topical application of coenzyme Q_{10} on adult periodontitis. *Mol Aspects Med* 15(Suppl.): S241–S248, 1994.

2. Iwamoto Y, Watanabe T, Okamoto H, et al. Clinical effect of coenzyme Q_{10} on periodontal disease. As cited in Folkers K, Yamamura Y, eds. Biomedical & clinical aspects of coenzyme Q_{10}, Vol 3. Amsterdam: Elsevier/North-Holland Biomedical Press, 1981: 109–119.

3. Folkers K and Yamamura Y. Biomedical and clinical aspects of coenzyme Q_{10}, Vol. 1. Amsterdam: Elsevier/North-Holland Biomedical Press, 1977: 294–311.

4. Wilkinson EG, Arnold RM, and Folkers K. Treatment of periodontal and other soft tissue diseases of the oral cavity with coenzyme Q_{10}. As cited in Folkers K, Yamamura Y, eds. Biomedical & clinical aspects of coenzyme Q_{10}, Vol. 1. Amsterdam: Elsevier/North-Holland Biomedical Press, 1977.

5. Wilkinson EG, Arnold RM, and Folkers K. Bioenergetics and clinical medicine. VI. Adjunctive treatment of periodontal disease with coenzyme Q_{10}. *Res Commun Chem Pathol Pharmacol* 14(4): 715–719, 1976.

6. Littarru G, et al. Deficiency of coenzyme Q_{10} in gingival tissue from patients with periodontal disease. *Proc Natl Acad Sci USA* 68(10): 2332–2335, 1971.

7. Iwamoto Y, Watanabe T, Okamoto H, et al., 1981.

8. Pack ARC. Folate mouthwash: Effects on established gingivitis in periodontal patients. *J Clin Periodontol* 11: 619–628, 1984.

9. Thomson ME and Pack ARC. Effects of extended systemic and topical folate supplementation on gingivitis of pregnancy. *J Clin Periodontol* 9(3): 275–280, 1982.

10. Pack ARC and Thomson ME. Effects of topical and systemic folic acid supplementation on gingivitis in pregnancy. *J Clin Periodontol* 7(5): 402–414, 1980.

11. Vogel RI, et al. The effect of topical application of folic acid on gingival health. *J Oral Med* 33(1): 20–22, 1978.

Premenstrual Stress Syndrome

1. Thys-Jacobs S, et al. Calcium carbonate and the premenstrual syndrome: Effects on premenstrual and menstrual symptoms. *Am J Ob Gyn* 179(2): 444–452, 1998.

2. Alvir JM and Thys-Jacobs S. Premenstrual and menstrual symptom clusters and response to calcium treatment. *Psychopharmacol Bull* 27(2): 145–148, 1991.

3. Thys-Jacobs S, Ceccarelli S, Bierman A, et al. Calcium supplementation in premenstrual syndrome: A randomized crossover trial. *J Gen Intern Med* 4(3): 183–189, 1989.

4. Milewicz A, et al. *Vitex agnus-castus* extract in the treatment of luteal phase defects due to latent hyperprolactinemia. Results of a randomized placebo-controlled double-blind study. *Arzneimittelforschung* 43(7): 752–756, 1993.

5. Jarry H, et al. In vitro prolactin but not LH and FSH release is inhibited by compounds in extracts of *Agnus-castus*: direct evidence for a dopaminergic principle by the dopamine receptor assay. *EYP Clin Endocrinol* 102: 448–454, 1994.

6. Sliuz G, et al. *Agnus-castus* extracts inhibit prolactin secretion of rat pituitary cells. *Horm Metab Res* 25(5): 253–255, 1993.

7. Schulz V, et al. Rational phytotherapy. New York: Springer-Verlag, 1998: 241–242.

8. Dittmar FW, et al. Premenstrual syndrome: Treatment with a phytopharmaceutical. *Therapiewoche Gynakol* 5: 60–68, 1992.

9. Peteres-Welte C, et al. Menstrual abnormalities and PMS: *Vitex agnus-castus*. *Therapiewoche Gynakol* 7: 49–52, 1994.

10. Coeugniet E, et al. Premenstrual syndrome (PMS) and its treatment. *Arztezeitschr Naturheilverf* 27: 619–622, 1986.

11. Lauritzen C, et al. Treatment of premenstrual tension syndrome with *Vitex agnus-castus*. Controlled, double-blind study vs. pyridoxine. *Phytomedicine* 4(3): 183–189, 1997.

12. Lauritzen C, et al., 1997.

13. Schulz V, et al., 1998: 243.

14. Cahill DJ, et al. Multiple follicular development associated with herbal medicine. *Hum Reprod* 9(8): 1469–1470, 1994.

15. Propping D, et al. *Agnus-castus*: treatment of gynaecological syndromes. *Theapeutikon* 5(110): 581–585, 1991.

16. Diegoli MS, et al. A double-blind trial of four medications to treat severe premenstrual syndrome. *Int J Gynaecol Obstet* 62: 63–67, 1998.

17. Kleijnen J, Ter Riet G, and Knipschild P. Vitamin B_6 in the treatment of premenstrual syndrome—a review. *Br J Obstet Gynaecol* 97(9): 847–852, 1990.

18. London RS, et al. Efficacy of alpha-tocopherol in the treatment of the premenstrual syndrome. *J Reprod Med* 32(6): 400–404, 1987.

19. Facchinetti F, Bolrella P, Sances G, et al. Oral magnesium successfully relieves premenstrual mood changes. *Obstet Gynecol* 78(2): 177–181, 1991.

20. Facchinetti F, et al. Magnesium prophylaxis of menstrual migraine: effects on intracellular magnesium. *Headache* 31: 298–304, 1991.

21. London RS, Bradley L, and Chiamori NY. Effect of a nutritional supplement on premenstrual symptomatology in women with premenstrual syndrome: a double-blind longitudinal study. *J Am Coll Nutr* 10(5): 494–499, 1991.

22. Reynolds MA and London RS. Efficacy of a multivitamin/mineral supplement in the treatment of the premenstrual syndrome (Abstract). *J Am Coll Nutr* 7(5): 416, 1988.

23. Stewart A. Clinical and biochemical effects of nutritional supplementation on the premenstrual syndrome. *J Reprod Med* 32(6): 435–441, 1987.

24. Chakmakjian ZH, Higgins CE, and Abraham GE. The effect of a nutritional supplement, Optivite for Women, on premenstrual tension syndromes: II. Effect on symptomatology, using a double-blind, cross-over design. *J Appl Nutr* 37(1): 12–17, 1985.

25. Puolakka J, et al. Biochemical and clinical effects of treating the premenstrual syndrome with prostaglandin synthesis precursors. *J Reprod Med* 30: 149–153, 1985.

26. Dittmar FW, et al., 1992.

Psoriasis

1. Bittiner SB, et al. A double-blind, randomised, placebo-controlled trial of fish oil in psoriasis. *Lancet* i: 378–380, 1988.

2. Soyland E, Funk J, Rajka G, et al. Effect of dietary supplementation with very-long-chain n-3 fatty acids in patients with psoriasis. *N Engl J Med* 328: 1812–1816, 1993.

Raynaud's Disease

1. Sunderland GT, Belch JJF, Sturrock RD, et al. A double-blind randomised placebo controlled trial of Hexopal in primary Raynaud's disease. *Clin Rheumatol* 7(1): 46–49, 1988.

2. DiGiacomo RA, Kremer JM, and Shah DM. Fish-oil dietary supplementation in patients with Raynaud's phenomenon: a double-blind, controlled, prospective study. *Am J Med* 86: 158–164, 1989.

3. Ringer TV, et al. Fish oil blunts the pain response to cold pressor testing in normal males (Abstract). *J Am Coll Nutr* 8(5): 435, 1989.

4. Belch JJF, et al. Evening primrose oil (Efamol) as a treatment for cold-induced vasospasm (Raynaud's phenomenon). *Prog Lipid Res* 25: 335–340, 1986.

5. Belch JJF, et al. Evening primrose oil (Efamol) in the treatment of Raynaud's phenomenon: A double-blind study. *Thromb Haemost* 54(2): 490–494, 1985.

6. Jung F, et al. Effect of *Ginkgo biloba* on fluidity of blood and peripheral microcirculation in volunteers. *Arzneimittelforschung Drug Res* 40: 589–593, 1990.

Rheumatoid Arthritis

1. James MJ, et al. Dietary n-3 fatty acids and therapy for rheumatoid arthritis. *Semin Arthr Rheum* 27: 85–97, 1997.

2. Harris WS. Dietary fish oil and blood lipids. *Curr Opin Lipidol* 7: 3–7, 1996.

3. Harris WS. Fish oils and plasma lipid and lipoprotein metabolism in humans: a critical review. *J Lipid Res* 30: 785–807, 1989.

4. Cobiac L, Clifton PM, and Abbey M. Lipid, lipoprotein, and hemostatic effects of fish vs. fish-oil n-3 fatty acids in mildly hyperlipidemic males. *Am J Clin Nutr* 53: 1210–1216, 1991.

5. Harris WS. n-3 Fatty acids and serum lipoproteins: human studies. *Am J Clin Nutr* 65(suppl.): 1645S–1654S, 1997.

6. Shapiro JA, Koepsell TD, Voight LF, et al. Diet and rheumatoid arthritis in women: a possible protective effect of fish consumption. *Epidemiology* 7: 256–263, 1996.

7. Singh GB and Atal CK. Pharmacology of an extract of salai guggal ex-*Boswellia serrata*, a new non-steroidal anti-inflammatory agent. *Agents Action* 18: 407–412, 1986.

8. Wildfeuer A, Neu IS, Safayhi H, et al. Effects of boswellic acids extracted from an herbal medicine on the biosynethsis of leukotrienes and the course of experimental autoimmune encephalomyelitis. *Arzneimittelforschung* 48(6): 668–674, 1998.

9. Etzel R. Special extract of *Boswellia serrata* in the treatment of rheumatoid arthritis. *Phytomedicine* 3(1): 67–70, 1996.

10. Sander O, Herborn G, and Rau R. Is H15 (resin extract of *Boswellia serrata*, "incense") a useful supplement to established drug therapy of chronic polyarthritis? Results of a double-blind pilot study (Eng Abst Only). *Z Rheumatol* 57(1): 11–16, 1998.

11. ESCOP monographs. Fascicule 2: *Harpagophyti radix* (devil's claw). Exeter, UK: European Scientific Cooperative on Phytotherapy, 1997: 5.

12. ESCOP monographs, 1997: 4

13. ESCOP monographs, 1997: 5.

14. ESCOP monographs, 1997: 4.

15. Satoskar RR, et al. Evaluation of anti-inflammatory property of curcumin diferuloyl methane. *Ind J Med Res* 71: 632–634, 1980.

16. Deodhar SD, et al. Preliminary studies on antirheumatic activity of curcumin. *Ind J Med Res* 71: 632–634, 1980.

17. Schulz V, et al. Rational phytotherapy. New York: Springer-Verlag, 1998: 263.

18. Ammon HPT, et al. Pharmacology of *Curcuma longa*. *Planta Medica* 57: 1–7, 1991.

19. Bingham R, et al. Yucca plant saponin in the management of arthritis. *J Appl Nutr* 27: 45–50, 1975.

20. Zurier RB, et al. Gamma-linolenic acid treatment of rheumatoid arthritis: A randomized, placebo-controlled trial. *Arthritis Rheum* 39(11): 1808–1817, 1996.

21. Peretz A, et al. Adjuvant treatment of recent onset rheumatoid arthritis by selenium supplementation: preliminary observations. *Br J Rheumatol* 31: 281–286, 1992.

22. Tarp U, et al. Selenium treatment in rheumatoid arthritis. *Acta Pharmacol Toxicol* 59(Suppl. 7): 382–385, 1986.

23. Tarp U, et al. Selenium treatment in rheumatoid arthritis. *Scand J Rheumatol* 14(4): 364–368, 1985.

24. Peretz A, et al. Zinc distribution in blood components, inflammatory status, and clinical indexes of disease activity during zinc supplementation in inflammatory rheumatic diseases. *Am J Clin Nutr* 57: 690–694, 1993.

25. Rasker JJ and Kardaun SH. Lack of beneficial effect of zinc sulphate in rheumatoid arthritis. *Scand J Rheumatol* 11: 168–170, 1982.

26. Simkin PA. Treatment of rheumatoid arthritis with oral zinc sulfate. *Agents Actions* 8(Suppl.): 587–596, 1981.

27. Darlington LG and Ramsey NW. Review of dietary therapy for rheumatoid arthritis. *Br J Rheumatol* 32(6): 507–514, 1993.

28. Kjeldsen-Kragh J. Controlled trial of fasting and one-year vegetarian diet in rheumatoid arthritis. *Lancet* 338(8772): 899–902, 1991.

29. Nenonen M, et al. Effects of uncooked vegan food "living food" on rheumatoid arthritis, a three month controlled and randomised study (Abstract). *Am J Clin Nutr* 56: 762, 1992.

Ulcers

1. Kassir ZA. Endoscopic controlled trial of four drug regimens in the treatment of chronic duodenal ulceration. *Irish Med J* 78: 153–156, 1985.

2. Morgan AG, et al. Comparison between cimetidine and Caved-S in the treatment of gastric ulceration and subsequent maintenance therapy. *Gut* 23: 545–551, 1982.

3. Morgan AG, et al. Maintenance therapy: A two year comparison between Caved-S and cimetidine treatment in the prevention of symptomatic gastric ulcer. *Gut* 26: 599–602, 1985.

4. Murray M and Pizzorno J. Encyclopedia of natural medicine, 2nd ed. Rocklin, CA: Prima Publishing, 1997: 815.

5. Murray M and Pizzorno J, 1997.

6. Beil W, et al. Effects of flavonoids on parietal cell acid secretion, gastric mucosal prostaglandin production and *Helicobacter pylori* growth. *Arzneimittelforschung Drug Res* 45: 697–700, 1995.

Varicose Veins

1. Schulz V, et al. Rational phytotherapy. New York: Springer-Verlag, 1998: 131–134.

2. Neiss A, et al. Zum Wirksamkeitsnachweis von Rosskastaniensamenextrakt beim varikosen Symptomenkomplex. *Munch Med Wochenschr* 7: 213–216, 1976.

3. Diehm C, et al. Comparison of leg compression stocking and oral horse-chestnut seed extract therapy in patients with chronic venous insufficiency. *Lancet* 347: 292–294, 1996.

4. Kreysel HW, et al. A possible role of lysosomal enzymes in the pathogenesis of varicocosis and the reduction in their serum activity by Venostatin®. *Vasa* 12: 377–382, 1983.

5. Schulz V, et al., 1998: 131.

6. Newall C, et al. Herbal medicines: a guide for health-care professionals. London: The Pharmaceutical Press, 1996: 166–167.

7. Schulz V, et al., 1998: 132.

8. Schwitters B, et al. OPC in practice: Bioflavanols and their applications. Rome: Alfa Omega, 1993.

9. Masquelier J, et al. Stabilization of collagen by procyanidolic oligomers. *Acta Ther* 7: 101–105, 1981.

10. Masquelier J. Procyanidolic oligomers. *J Parums Cosm Arom* 95: 89–97, 1990.

11. Tixier JM, et al. Evidence by in vivo and in vitro studies that binding of pycnogenols to elastin affects its rate of degradation by elastases. *Biochem Pharmacol* 33: 3933–3939, 1984.

12. Bombardelli E, et al. *Vitis vinifera L. Fitoterapia* 66: 291–317, 1995.

13. Henriet JP. Exemplary study for a phlebotropic substance, the EIVE study. On file with Primary Services International, Southport, CT.

14. Delacroix P, et al. Double-blind study of endotelon in chronic venous insufficiency. La Revue de Medicine 31: 27–28, 1793–1802, 1981.

15. Bombardelli E, et al., 1995.

16. Schulz V, et al., Rational phytotherapy. New York: Springer-Verlag, 1998: 283.

17. Kartnig T. Clinical applications of *Centella asiatica* (L.) Urb. *Herbs Spices Med Plants* 3: 146–173, 1988.

18. Castellani C, et al. The *Centella asiatica*. *Boll Chim Farm* 120: 570–605, 1981.

19. Belcaro GV, et al. Capillary filtration and ankle edema in patients with venous hypertension treated with TTFCA. *Angiology* 41: 12–18, 1990.

20. Cesarone MR, et al. The microcirculatory activity of *Centella asiatica* in venous insufficiency: A double-blind study. *Minerva Cardioangiol* 42: 299–304, 1994.

21. Pointel JP, et al. Titrated extract of *Centella asiatica* (TECA) in the treatment of venous insufficiency of the lower limbs. *Angiology* 38: 46–50, 1987.

22. Cesarone MR, et al. Activity of *Centella asiatica* in venous insufficiency. *Minerva Cardioangiol* 42: 137–143, 1992.

23. Kartnig T., 1988.

24. Nalini K, et al. Effect of *Centella asiatica* fresh leaf aqueous extract on learning and memory and biogenic amine turnover in albino rats. *Fitoterapia* 63(3): 232–237, 1992.

25. Bosse JP, et al. Clinical study of a new antikeloid drug. *Ann Plast Surg* 3: 13–21, 1979.

26. Basellini A, et al. Varicose disease in pregnancy. *Ann Obstet Gyn Med Perinat* 106: 337–341, 1985.

27. Bone K. *Mediherb Professional Review* 59: 3, 1997.

28. Bone K., 1997.

29. Gabor M. Pharmacologic effects of flavonoids on blood vessels. *Angiologica* 9: 355–374, 1972.

30. Mian E, et al. Anthocyanosides and the walls of microvessels: Further aspects of the mechanism of action of their protective effect in syndromes due to abnormal capillary fragility. *Minerva Med* 68: 3565–3581, 1977.

31. Havsteen B. Flavonoids, a class of natural products of high pharmacological potency. *Biochem Pharmacol* 32: 1141–1148, 1983.

32. Lietti A, et al. Studies on *Vaccinium myrtillus* anthocyanosides. I. Vasoprotective and anti-inflammatory activity. *Arzneimittelforschung* 26: 829–832, 1976.

33. Eandi M. Unpublished results. As cited in Morazzoni P, et al. eds. *Vaccinium myrtillus*. *Fitoterapia* 67(1): 3–29, 1996.

34. Petruzezellis V, et al. Therapeutic action of oral doses of mesoglycan in the pharmacological treatment of varicose syndrome and its complications. *Minerva Med* 76: 543–548, 1985.

35. Sangrigoli V. Mesoglycan in acute and chronic venous insufficiency of the legs. *Clin Ther* 129(3): 207–209, 1989.

36. Oddone G, et al. Assessment of the effects of oral mesoglycan sulphate in patients with chronic venous pathology of the lower extremities. *Gazzetta Medica Italiana* 146: 111–114, 1987.

Index

Note: The boldfaced terms are the principal natural treatments for the conditions under which they are listed.

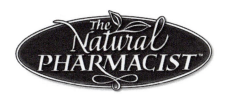

About the Series Editors

Steven Bratman, M.D., medical director of Prima Health, has many years of experience in the alternative medicine field. A graduate of the University of California at Davis, Medical School, he has also trained in herbology, nutrition, Chinese medicine, and other alternative therapies, and has worked closely with a wide variety of alternative practitioners. He is the author of *The Natural Pharmacist: Your Complete Guide to Herbs* (Prima), *The Natural Pharmacist Guide to St. John's Wort and Depression* (Prima), *The Alternative Medicine Ratings Guide* (Prima), and *The Alternative Medicine Sourcebook* (Lowell House).

David J. Kroll, Ph.D., is a professor of pharmacology and toxicology at the University of Colorado School of Pharmacy and a consultant for pharmacists, physicians, and alternative practitioners on the indications and cautions for herbal medicine use. A graduate of both the University of Florida and the Philadelphia College of Pharmacy and Science, Dr. Kroll has lectured widely and has published articles in a number of medical journals, abstracts, and newsletters.